KINKY HISTORY

KINKY HISTORY

A Rollicking Journey through
Our Sexual Past, Present, and Future

ESMÉ LOUISE JAMES

WITH DR. SUSAN JAMES

A TarcherPerigee Book

tarcherperigee

an imprint of Penguin Random House LLC
penguinrandomhouse.com

Most TarcherPerigee books are available at special quantity discounts for bulk purchase for sales promotions,
premiums, fund-raising, and educational needs. Special books or book excerpts also can be created to fit
specific needs. For details, write: SpecialMarkets@penguinrandomhouse.com.

Library of Congress Cataloging-in-Publication Data

Names: James, Esmé Louise, author.
Title: Kinky history: a rollicking journey through our sexual past, present, and future / Esmé Louise James.
Description: New York: TarcherPerigee, Penguin Random House LLC, [2024] | Includes index.
Identifiers: LCCN 2023044485 (print) | LCCN 2023044486 (ebook) |
ISBN 9780593716908 (hardcover) | ISBN 9780593716915 (epub)
Subjects: LCSH: Sex—History. | Homosexuality—History. | Gender-nonconforming people—History.
Classification: LCC HQ12.J34 2024 (print) | LCC HQ12 (ebook) | DDC 306.709—dc23/eng/20231019
LC record available at https://lccn.loc.gov/2023044485
LC ebook record available at https://lccn.loc.gov/2023044486

Printed in the United States of America
1st Printing

Book design by Shannon Nicole Plunkett

For anyone who has ever searched for an open door when they needed a safe place to turn, who has ever felt alone and in need of a place to belong, who has ever been left unheard and wanted good company to understand them.

You are always welcome here.

A good dinner is of great importance to good talk.
One cannot think well, love well, sleep well,
if one has not dined well.

—Virginia Woolf, *A Room of One's Own*

Contents

Foreplay

I t is a truth universally acknowledged that we must hesitantly speak of the act that brought us all into this world. I must here ask you, gentle reader, to go no further if you are faint of heart, if you are endowed with that delicate sensitivity that makes improper conversation so insufferable to the nerves, for I am about to say an immodest word . . .

Sex.

Pick yourself up off the floor, I implore you! Let the breath return to your lungs. Allow your shaken nerves to settle, for I am bound to say many more such shocking things.

Shall we get some more out of the way?

Asshole. Vulva. Cock ring. Dildo.

These are the kinds of brazen words you may expect to see if you dare to read much further.

Sex is not a topic to be broached in polite conversation. However, I have always been of the opinion that the best parties are the ones that throw propriety out the window. And so, *shoo!* Off with you! Leave me the libertines, the ragbags, the artists, the figures of the night.

The purpose of this book is as simple as this: it is a conversation. It is a conversation that not only brings up impolite topics such as dildos (*gasp!*), orgasms (*shock!*), and anal (*horror!*), but it does so with a variety of colorful figures around the table. I have invited the past and present to join our discussion, and they have brought their painters, their radical thinkers, their politicians, their statisticians.

Sit with Aristotle as he philosophizes and soliloquizes, enjoying his "lesbian wine." Drink and be merry with Victor Hugo while he teaches us about the secret nightlife of Paris. Meet Gertrude Stein, who invented and reclaimed queer language; watch Albert Einstein condemn the unnatural constraints of marriage and James Joyce celebrate the beauty of his wife's farts; and admire Julius Caesar as he celebrates the joys of being a power bottom. We'll meet F. Scott Fitzgerald and Christian Grey, Jean-Jacques Rousseau and Hans Christian Andersen—and what kind of party would it be if Sigmund Freud and the Marquis de Sade did not make appearances?

Come and dine with all your favorite historical figures, and perhaps some with whom you have yet to become acquainted. (Have you met Alfred Kinsey or Theresa Berkley, Pietro Aretino or Richard von Krafft-Ebing?) Who knows who else may waltz in here? It is sure to be a lively crowd.

Did I tell you Mozart has composed a particularly dirty ditty for the evening?

It is going to be a noisy party, one that will be difficult to forget. I intend to record—with as much accuracy as multiple bottles of wine will allow—the dialogue that transpires between these voices: their arguments and debates, along with their sometimes surprising harmony of opinion.

A Note of Introduction

You may well ask what gives me the right to chair such a dynamic dinner table. What kind of host would I be if I didn't take a moment to properly introduce myself? I am, I imagine, no different from you—a curious mind who has often been bemused by the multilayered enigma of our sexuality. But where most would quite logically stop exploring these questions and return, respectfully, to their lives, I have decided to dedicate mine to studying prehistoric penises and pornography used at ancient orgies.

Questions about human sexuality have held me under their seductive spell for as long as I can remember. For the most part, these questions and conversations were all rooted in the present—until the day I was posed a question that would completely alter the course of my life. Picture in your mind, dear reader, an arts-major undergraduate student, fully equipped with almond latte and box-dyed red hair. I had come to university to study the history of religion. It was at this time of bright-eyed learning and painfully experimental drama productions that I was asked a life-changing question: Would I write a piece on the history of the dildo for a student magazine?

The *history* of the dildo? I mulled it over while I ate a discounted plate of tofu scramble. I had written plenty about dildos before this—I was approached for the job primarily because every piece I'd published up to that point had come with a sexual-content warning—but I'd never considered that they may have any kind of substantial history. So I did what any freelance writer would do when baffled by a brief—I went to Google.

BOOM! Out it poured, like a horny Pandora's box that had finally been jerked open. Prehistoric dildos, ancient strap-ons, jade butt plugs, and thirteenth-century cock rings made from the eyelids of goats. My obsession began. Sure, I'd known that humans must have fucked before us—otherwise we would have had a pretty slim chance of being here—but *surely* all the *kinky* stuff was novel to us? We were living in an age of liberation, daring to sexually experiment where no one had sexually experimented before. How could the use of sex toys be seen as radical today if we were using them back in the prehistoric era? How could fetishes be so shocking if we were already idolizing feet back in Aristotle's day?

A new world opened to me—a world I have come to call Kinky History.

This world may now be part of your world as well. I was sitting alone in lockdown, nursing a bottle of sparkling wine, when I decided to bring these stories into the digital sphere. Until then, my discoveries had remained limited to small publications and as icebreakers at parties (to which I was unlikely to get invited back). It was really the absence of being able to share what I had learned with friends, family, and peers that drew me to TikTok. I hadn't thought much about the reach my videos would have—and I certainly didn't envision having a following of over 2.5 million people from around the globe two years later. It was just going to be a way to share facts that had shocked me with the small group of people who would care.

From one slightly alcohol-induced video emerged a tiny community. I excitedly texted my best friend that twenty-six people had started following me! Their questions and comments inspired me to make another sixty-second video. They were all eager to learn more about the history of the dildo.

It came as a great surprise that what interested me could possibly interest anyone else. Within the first month, I was met with a pleasantly humbling realization: I wasn't special. The questions that fascinated me, the stories that captivated me, also held this power over thousands upon thousands of others. These were tales missing from mainstream history classes; these were facts about being human that were absent from our conversations. Sex and sexuality are a global topic of conversation, now more than ever before. Sex is, in many ways, a universal language that can transcend speech and cultural barriers, even if it is—as we will see throughout this book—very much defined by those forces.

Stuck in a one-bedroom city apartment, I would wait for my partner's Zoom meetings to finish before recording my lessons in the same room. I was incredibly fortunate to have a university friend I could reach out to as I entered this brave new world: Mary McGillivray (@_TheIconoclass) was teaching art history lessons to big audiences on TikTok, and as a testament to her character, she was always there to answer my elementary questions about video editing. It was because of the people around me that I became confident enough to take this seriously; to buy a microphone and better camera, to teach myself video editing and how to photoshop. It was from these humble origins that a community began to grow—a community that cared less about my early cringeworthy use of video effects and more about what I had to say.

Social media is an unpredictable beast, and there is no way to tell what stories will change your entire life overnight. One day, overcome by a sense of annoyance while writing my thesis, I picked up my phone to rant about the misconception that pornography is a new phenomenon, giving a list of pornographic novels from the 1600s to 1800s and calling this the "golden era of porn." I put down my phone, drove off for a doctor's appointment, and thought nothing more about it—until I was sitting in the waiting room watching my community grow thousands of people by the minute.

Kinky History was no longer just an outlet for my compulsive need to overshare; it had become a community of curious minds. Without meaning to, I had stumbled upon the true privilege of sharing and teaching these incredible tales of humans past. And the rest, as they say, is history.

A Note on Table Manners

I have saved one important seat at our table. Please, pour yourself a drink and enjoy the occasion. Come, kinksters and academics, critics and questioners. Something different has brought each of you to this table tonight. Whether it's a lifelong love of history or an impulsive decision to learn something new—whether you will be combing my words with a critical red pen or have merely found yourself aroused by the brightly lettered *KINKY* on the front cover—this is a safe space, and all are welcome here.

Participate in this conversation in the way that feels right to you. Feel free to laugh at the mention of penises (I highly encourage you to doodle some doodles in the margin whenever something particularly tickles your fancy), to take notes on points you would most like to remember, to furiously contend with me and passionately correct me (I have been on social media long enough to have seen it all), to further a story of interest with an analogy of your own, and to dog-ear the pages of any passage that has resonated with you. I am all ears.

One of the things that have always drawn me to books is the fact that they are participatory. As much as we authors like to flatter ourselves, only half of the encounter is owed to us. The rest comes from you, mysterious reader, and the qualities with which you will imbue my words. It comes from your imagination and your backstory, your expectations and your bias, your knowledge and your desires. Your experience at this dinner party will be truly unique from that of each of my other guests. Let us revel in that difference and celebrate its multiplicity. How wonderful is that?

Now, as you pass the threshold, please hang up your coat and hat. The one thing I ask is that you let go of any hesitation, expectations, and prejudices that may keep you waiting on the footpath. Enter with an open mind. We are going to be busting many myths. We are going to be calling many "commonly known facts" into question. We are going to be breaking glass, throwing plates around, and generally reveling in all kinds of deviance.

Let yourself be surprised. Be ready to recognize any preconceptions as they arise for you—I'm sure they will, as they have many a time for me. Be willing to question from where those preconceptions may have originated, and whether they are worth picking up again as you go back out into the world. It's in this space of openness, curiosity, and vulnerability that we permit ourselves the most profound revelations.

There is power in our silence, in our shrouds of secrecy. We have dressed sex up in rouge and fine lace, setting the imagination alight as it dreams of what remains concealed, curiosity turning to craving as we yearn for what we can't see. There is power in this secrecy—but it is not ours. We pedestalize something that was ours to begin with; we make dangerously unreachable something that was always meant to be touched.

What happens when we start to speak?

Isn't it strange, after all, that the thing that has remained so absent from our history books is the reason we have a history at all? That the essential act that connects us all has been, and continues to be, the source of so much division? Out of our basic needs—such as food, shelter, and water—how has one come to be shrouded in taboo? And even when we can bring it up, there are unspoken (though strictly enforced) rules for the conversation: what is classified as crude and what is educational; when it is inappropriate to keep talking; in whose company it is acceptable to discuss such matters.

Perhaps it is time we accept how impoverished our dialogue and understanding of history has been as a result of our failure to mention the very things that have brought it about—namely sex, gender, and identity. By refusing to let sex remain veiled in mystery, we take the power back. Sex is no longer an abstract construct we fear to touch but something that is tangible, bodily, felt—the way it was always meant to be.

Our conversation of sex and sexuality, gender and identity is far from a closed book. It is but one more chapter in a long-evolving discussion that has taken place throughout human history. And in the same way that these voices from the past continue to inform our present, I hope this conversation will join and expand the chorus.

Tasting Menu

By its very nature, any attempted history of these topics is going to be partial and contingent. They are such highly contested subjects, before even introducing the challenges associated with studying history itself. It is a pot of mysterious ingredients all mixed together without any traditional menu to guide us. More than with any other history book, an attempt to cover sex history is bound to be filled with rich and unpredictable flavors. We will be beginning from this place of paradox, finding our way through the menu with each bite and new taste that inspires us.

I have placed these dishes in an order that I believe best does justice to their tastes and textures. This is a subjective endeavor. It would be impossible to say that the dishes I have chosen, and the aperitives that go with them, are removed from my personal preferences. I have made cuts and additions, paired thoughts with wine, and taken dishes back to the kitchen to reseason and tweak or eliminate from the menu. I have done it all to inspire the conversation I believe we should be having around this table. The flavor combinations will not be to everyone's taste, but all I ask is that you take your seat with an explorative palate and allow yourself the opportunity to try something different.

Each of the five courses is organized around a theme that informs our sexual behavior to this day. We will begin with an exploration of sin, that fraught religious concept that has shaped our sex lives and intimate relationships in unexpected ways. Moving on to our next dish—one I intend to dwell on as long as possible—we will investigate self-pleasure. Next, we'll delve into the realm of gender identity and sexuality, tracing the questions and "queeries" that have pervaded our history. As the night draws on, we will try some more experimental flavors by exploring kinks and fetishes, tastes bound to disrupt the conceptions of sex we have hitherto established. We will finish the night with a bang, looking to one of the most contentious subjects in contemporary discussions about sexuality: pornography, and how it both has been shaped by and continues to shape our social world.

As I have mentioned, there are biases to be found in the study of history itself, to which sexual history is no exception. So much of recorded history (especially the further we reach back) is associated with Western civilizations. It has largely been shaped by dominant power structures such as capitalism, colonialism, patriarchy, and heteronormativity, and we must always remember that "history is written by victors." Stories that disrupt the dominant narrative have far too often been left on the cutting room floor of prominent historians, leaving others to scrounge around in these scraps hundreds of years later for indications of what might also have been. However, the collective result of these efforts is that we have found far too many missing, hidden, and partially revealed pieces to not call into question what these dominant narratives may otherwise have had us believe.

With each new piece, each new fragment, we have begun to tell a new story—a story that once again features the true variety of figures and facts that previously existed only in margins and shadows, unexplained references and neglected phrases. There is great power in finally telling and reclaiming these stories—if there weren't, they wouldn't have been suppressed in the first place.

To counter the Western frame my own education sets around this book, I have sought to recognize Eastern and First Nations cultures wherever possible and appropriate in my examples and stories, providing alternative points of view and diversity of thought and language with which to unpack these topics. Where these views and tales are no longer my place to speak about, I have pointed you toward alternative dinner parties that are better placed to host that conversation. I hope this is another step toward a future conversation that is far more diverse and inclusive.

A Special Guest

Despite what my delusions of grandeur would have me believe, I am not an expert in all things. This is why I have asked so many voices to join us here tonight, to share their wisdom and to arouse your imagination. We are greatly indebted to the minds that came before us in ways that can be quite impossible to perceive. None of these stories would have ever reached me if not for the academics who found them, the writers who have kept them alive, artists inspired by them, and critics who sought to question them. These tales are yours as much as they are mine. This conversation is as unfettered and free-flowing as any good dinner party should be.

There is one particular guest I do want to make special mention of. Allow me to introduce you to my mum.

When I first sat down to organize this dinner party, I wasn't sure how I would incorporate the present day into my dishes. I have spent so long in books and archives; I am far more acquainted with the Woolfs and Aquinases than I am with the equally formidable contributors of today. This is where my mum, Dr. Susan James, comes in. She can do something I could only hope, in my wildest dreams, to do—she can do math. In math class, I was always more interested in why the observer had stopped to admire the tree from a particular angle rather than working out what that angle was. As a result, I found myself ill-equipped to understand and do justice to contemporary research surrounding gender, identity, and sexuality.

As Kinky History was blowing up in 2021, my mum—a formidable mathematician and statistician who will forever question how she lost her daughter to the study of history—suggested I expand my series to incorporate recent statistical research.

"I wouldn't know the first place to begin!" I exclaimed, trapped in flashbacks of working out how many apples Tommy would have left if Miranda took eight. Who needs that many apples anyway?

"You can start right here," Mum declared, dumping a pile of research papers, all highlighted and annotated in true *Dummies' Guide* fashion, on the table.

In an emerging pattern with most of my life-changing moments, we proceeded to open a bottle of sparkling wine, and the idea of SexTistics was born—a documentary series using statistics to provide a snapshot of our intimate lives, combining our respective knowledge and skills to erase the taboo that still exists around this information.

I will resist saying here "and the rest was history," because it is very much of the present. It was from the combined efforts of Kinky History and SexTistics that this book was created. It is with the help of my cohost that we have been able to lay the present day proudly on the table among the historical dishes, and with it such figures as Alfred Kinsey, William H. Masters and Virginia E. Johnson, and Katharine Davis, modern sex researchers. We have been able to identify contemporary trends and place them against the ebbs and flows in historical cycles. We have been able to construct our historical narrative through numbers, bringing the past into closer conversation with our world today.

Most important, this effort has allowed greater space for *you*. As part of our project, we sent out a survey about sexual identity and behavior through our social media networks. We received responses from over one hundred different countries (most coming from the United States, Australia, the United Kingdom, and Canada). With the ongoing impact of the pandemic, innumerable research studies have remained on hold, especially those on a larger scale. When it comes to statistics, even the most recent national surveys surrounding relationships, sex, and gender are now outdated, with the last studies in the US, Australia, and the UK now all nearly a decade old.

Our main reason for conducting this survey—with comparable numbers to those in previous national surveys—was to ensure that the conversation would not be outdated before it even began. By placing our results against those of the studies completed nearly ten years ago, we can also give an insight into how quickly thinking about sex, identity, and gender has shifted, further emphasizing the importance of having this conversation right now.

Our survey does not come without its own biases. People who responded were largely existing followers of Kinky History and/or SexTistics, meaning that many likely thought liberally about sex (you saucy devils); 67.5 percent identified as female. We included options for nonbinary, trans men and women, and "other" in our gender categorization—allowing us to include the experience of people who, in far too many cases, have been placed into the "too hard" category and disregarded.

Our respondents also skewed to the younger generations, 67.3 percent of participants being between twenty and thirty-nine years old. Equally, there was a large proportion with a higher level of education, with nearly 61.1 percent having a post–high school education, and 37.1 percent having either an undergraduate or postgraduate degree. As we will see once we make our way to the third course, "Queer Kinks," the dominance of this younger generation with advanced degrees may account for the large number of participants who classified themselves as queer. For instance, the proportion of people identifying as bisexual on our survey was 33.8 percent—nearly as many as those who identified as homosexual (39.3 percent). All these factors will come into play as we discuss our results. And for my STEM-inclined readers who love to dig into the numbers, a fuller picture of the data we collected can be found as an appendix at the back of this book.

This all being said, it does not mean our survey should be discarded as a product of the #LeftistAgenda. The large sample size (14,058 participants), as well as the comparable results it has produced, means it's not to be scoffed at. The study of statistics is all about the quality of the data you produce and your ability to interpret it in a meaningful way. I know that my mum has provided excellent data and interpreted it perfectly.

Like words and language, numbers are also open to interpretation. And as scary as this prospect can be, it is also part of their appeal. The stories these numbers can tell us may lead us to make so many fascinating and unpredictable conclusions—conclusions that continue to challenge our received wisdom about sex.

A Matter of Housekeeping

Before we begin both dinner and conversation—the latter filled with Fleshlights, leather harnesses, erotic furniture, and more—it is worth pausing to reflect on one question: What exactly *is* sex? This subject, which has gathered such an assortment of people around the table tonight, is nebulous. How do we categorize it? What is its formal definition? Can it be removed from physicality or is it firmly rooted in the acts of the body?

Sex can have many definitions, and any study of it must embrace this ambiguity. Contrary to what some intoxicated figures around a bar may have you believe, our understanding of the subject is far more complicated than simply scoring a goal in a hole. A true enigma, it can appear to us in a variety of manifestations: sex as an impulse, a yearning, a sensation. We may talk about *sexual desire*: a drive to engage in or seek out sexual activities. We may speak about *sexual behavior*—which, in many cases, is the physical expression of this desire. We may speak about *sexual identity*: how an individual thinks about themselves in terms of who and even what they sexually desire.

None of these definitions remain stagnant. Indeed, we will find that each definition of sex will bring with it far more questions than answers. Does desire need to be physically consummated before it can be considered sexual? What kind of sexual behavior can be classified as sex? What distinguishes the act of sex from foreplay? What distinguishes sexual from romantic attraction, and at what stage do we consider preferences as part of one's identity, as opposed to a fleeting or occasional desire?

Following these questions as they arise can take us down enticing pathways. Nothing is guaranteed here; nothing is left unquestioned. We will follow the little white rabbit as far down as we can, until we reach our own realms of possibility. What can be found there and brought back to this world is entirely up to you. Our language around sexuality, sex, gender, and identity remains fervently contested because these concepts are difficult to capture in concise, universal, or final definitions. They are always changing, always subjective. Like the English language itself, these words have far more exceptions than they have rules. This is the tantalizing Wonderland we are about to enter.

When looking at gender, identity, and sexuality within history, it's important to remember that we are viewing it through a modern-day lens. The terminology we use today was not around in the times of many of the figures we will be discussing, and they are not here to confirm or deny the accuracy of our deductions. We can theorize whether these figures from the past may have been gay or bisexual, transgender or gender-nonconforming. In fact, I believe it is vital to do so, to demonstrate the long lineage of these communities. However, it is equally important to remember that we can never say for sure that these labels were the right fit for any of them.

Our understanding of the modern world is greatly affected by the way we tell history—for this reason, discussions of consent are as crucial in history as they are today. Self-expression looks different for everyone. So when we look back on those who came before us, I think it is far more important to pay attention to the means by which *they* chose to express *themselves* than it is to subject them to a contemporary understanding of identity that would be foreign to them. It is a bit of a paradox, isn't it? We're searching for communion with historical figures and movements to affirm our contemporary attitudes, even though language and understanding can differ so much across history and geography.

A Note on Kink

Indeed, you will find many such paradoxes in our conversation about sexual history this evening. I refer to these as the "kinks"— not kinky in a sexual sense, but kinks in terms of their other meaning: a twist or a curve in an otherwise straight line. These are the ideas that deviate from our norms and conventional wisdom, because, as you will see, the study of sexual history raises many conundrums, contradictions, ambiguities, and paradoxes for us to explore.

But here is a recommendation that might strike you as counterintuitive: it's better for us to sit with those kinks, and even to embrace and celebrate them, than to try to bend or stretch them into, ah, straightness. Humans are contradictory, messy creatures, and perhaps no aspect of our behaviors and identities better demonstrates that than our sexuality. Complications, contradictions, and ambiguity are a natural and even healthy part of our sexual lives—as they should be in sexual research and history. Indeed, there are many cautionary tales about what happens when we try to "iron out" those kinks—when we try to label, diagnose, and criminalize that which we don't understand. This is a risky and often downright dangerous exercise, one that has led to centuries of oppression and persecution for so many people.

We will encounter a number of tipping points—periods of truly significant, reverberating change—in this kinky historical timeline. They are the cumulative results of small and big alterations in our patterns of thinking, ones that may have built up over the course of decades or even centuries. Coming to understand the factors that led to historical tipping points helps us address stigmas today. We will come to understand that much of our inherited knowledge about sex doesn't comprise immutable facts, but rather that these are almost entirely culturally determined. Our thinking has changed time and time again, as thinkers and leaders introduced new lines of inquiry best suited to address the needs of their era.

I think I would be justified in declaring we are reaching a tipping point of our own. The topics of sexuality, identity, and gender have emerged from that "unspeakable" category they were boxed in, even in history as recent as my own childhood. Advances in the way we communicate have transformed this conversation. We are occupying a unique moment in history, with an immediacy of information like we have never seen before. Technological advancements, ecological crises, global pandemics, collectively traumatizing events—all of these factors have led to social and cultural change at a rate so rapid as to be barely comparable to that we have seen in the past. This has made it impossible to keep "impolite" conversations away. These topics are front and center in media coverage, with comment sections becoming a chorus of clashing opinions and debates. As Jane Smith (*It's wine o'clock somewhere!*) on Facebook will passionately tell you, everyone today is obsessed with sex and it's ruining our civilization.

If we are heading toward such a tipping point, it is worth stopping to ask ourselves: What is the new future that we want to see?

The answer lies in embracing these "kinks" in our thinking about sex and sexuality. Shall we raise a glass? Here's to interrogating issues of power and patriarchy, identity and social norms, empathy and vulnerability.

And now to the matter of events for the evening. Ensure that your dance card is left empty; there is a titillating variety of entertainment in store. Let your imagination and intellect be aroused by a range of impolite topics of conversation: the ancient origins of the dildo; the celebration and suppression of homoeroticism throughout history; the creation of the first pornographic novel and its threatened existence underground; bondage and sex toys, which soared in sales through the pandemic; masturbation and the shits we didn't give about it for the majority of history; *Fifty Shades of Grey*—fact or fiction?; and, of course, tentacle porn, and how it changed the world as we know it.

We will learn that nothing is new. Every single freaky inclination you've ever had has been with us for many hundreds of years, if not more. Humans have enjoyed being spanked and gagged, humiliated and worshipped, titillated and tortured since time immemorial. Nothing is new—only the names and paradigms through which we understand these things. Equipped with the right tools, we can look back into the past and uncover all the secrets that were always there, hidden for us to find. Like travelers to foreign lands, we will learn the languages and codes of these different times and places. And with a little luck, out from these dusty books will pour our libertines and licentious women, our artisans and our ass men, our cock rings and our condoms, our queens and our queers—the brilliant assortment that makes any party worth attending.

I am so happy you will be joining us this evening. Please make yourself right at home. I hope you will find something to make you laugh and to make you cry, to make you tug at the ends of your hair, or perhaps to plunge you into a state of existential contemplation. Enjoy the night in whatever way feels right to you.

It is now time to enter and take your place. Feel free to leave us and return again when you are ready; feel free to make yourself a regular guest. My door is always open, with warm dinner and company waiting. Pour yourself some wine, loosen your clothing, and make yourself comfortable.

Let's talk about sex.

THE SIN KINK

Follow me into the dining room. Please, find your seat and take a sip of the wine; you're going to need it. You will have time to become acquainted with everyone at this party, but first, there is a particular someone I would love you to meet.

I think I can hear his voice booming across the room . . .

Drink to the point of hilarity!

Ah, yes. There he is! Let's follow his advice and hear what else he has to say.

When I first became acquainted with Thomas Aquinas, he was a mythical creature not to be touched. He was ritually referenced at every church service and school assembly. It was not until my adolescence that this figure was given a body, made flesh by the hands of one influential teacher.

Once a year, the best and brightest students from local independent high schools were sent to a conference run by theologian Peter Vardy. This was by far my favorite day of the year. I was not brought up religious. My mum had been sent to a Catholic school just in case my grandparents were wrong for not believing in God. The school I attended, in a publicly performed existential crisis, removed "Anglican Christian School" from its name every second year and then put it back on.

It was, therefore, to both of my parents' shock that I asked for a Bible for my twelfth birthday. Specifically, I didn't want a Bible with pretty pictures and iconography; I wanted one with footnotes. Nothing intrigues me more than when I am told not to talk about something. The ambiguities and half-finished phrases

I encountered in school church services (when they were run, every second year) set my mind aflame—and my parents became the only ones to wish their child had just become obsessed with video games instead.

Aquinas, are you in here? Come and join us at the table.

I have encountered some fantastic teachers in my life, but Peter Vardy was one of the most influential. He riddled us about ethics and morals, introduced us to ancient philosophers and their theories. He didn't recite quotes without context, and he didn't dismiss Aquinas as an obscure presence in Christian history. He didn't only teach you about religion: he taught you to question it. He was unafraid to talk about the things we weren't meant to talk about. He taught us about the comfort food of saints, and that wombats have rectangular intestinal tracts so their poo is always shaped like a cube.* These facts are equally important.

After my first conference, I solidified myself as truly the Nerd of the Nerds, buying up every book of Vardy's available on the outside table. But there was one, pushed to the back and purposefully hidden, that really caught my attention. The book was called *The Puzzle of Sex*, and it was how I first truly made Aquinas's acquaintance.

Ah, there you are, Thomas. The glasses are full, so come meet our new guest.

---

* A silly factoid that has, unfortunately, been debunked in recent times.

The Invention of Innocence

In the thirteenth century, a man named Thomas Aquinas made a declaration that would influence our cultural worldview to this very day: the purpose of sex was procreation. Writing between the years 1265 and 1275 at the University of Paris, prominent Christian theologian Aquinas would be inspired by the translated works of Aristotle, which had only recently come to light. Quite ironically, Aristotle was highly skeptical of religious devotion; he most famously remarked, "Men create gods in their own image, not only with regard to their form but with regard to their mode of life." Even so, his ancient writings would shape the future of Christian thinking due to Aquinas's interpretation.

See, Aristotle had defined each aspect of human nature in terms of its purpose, down to the most nitty-gritty details. Things are "good" when they fulfill their purpose and things are "bad" when they fail to fulfill their purpose. A governor is good when they succeed at governing, just as a teacher is good when they succeed at educating. A set of legs is good if they succeed at walking, and a wombat's asshole is good if it produces cubic poos. Good things equate to happiness, and happiness is the purpose of life.

Besides the whole "Prayers and sacrifices to the gods are of no avail," Aquinas could get down with everything that Aristotle was saying. It was up to thinkers like himself to instruct others in how to lead a good life, and the ancient wisdom Aristotle had laid out did, indeed, seem pretty wise. Once the purpose of every aspect of human nature had been determined—a task that appeared more or less easy to do—there was a clear framework of "good" versus "bad" actions. Aquinas thus put forth the Natural Law, a foolproof guide to goodness, as, "All acts of virtue are prescribed by the Natural Law: since each one's reason naturally dictates to him to act virtuously." The various functions of human life and the body are determined through use of (his) reason—and when it came to genitalia, the sole purpose was determined to be reproduction.

As a result, any other use or function of genitalia thus becomes "intrinsically evil," as it is not fulfilling its purpose. This includes masturbation, oral sex, anal sex, same-sex encounters, and performing a puppet show using your penis, among others. (Though rarely mentioned in theological documents, penis puppetry really should be considered exceptionally bad.)

The Catholic Church accepted Aquinas's conception of sexual morality, and the enduring influence this has had, to the present day, is incalculable. The only purpose of sex was reproduction, and the only place for sex *or* reproduction was within the sacrament of marriage. Any other sex act, in any other context, was steeped in sin.

While this rule may seem clear-cut, there are inconsistencies and contradictions already appearing as cracks in the foundation. Peter Vardy laid out the assumptions that this line of thinking takes for granted:

1. That there is a single human nature that we all share.

2. That the purpose of genitalia is reproduction and, therefore, any use of genitalia for any other purpose is wrong.

3. That certain actions are "intrinsically evil"—wrong in and of themselves, without taking consequences or benefits into account.

There is also the contradiction between requiring adherence to a "natural law" and the fact that sex can only take place within the bounds of marriage—an institution that is not found in the laws of nature, but is peculiar to human civilization. The road map can therefore be summarized as such: humans should always act as nature prescribes, except when Christian traditions contradict these natural instincts (and then they should stick to those traditions instead).

This is the first historical tipping point we have encountered tonight—moments in which radical thoughts and movements have shaken the course of history so strongly that we are still feeling the reverberations of them today. The ripples of Aquinas's work are undoubtedly with us every time we talk about sex—just as the ripples of previous tipping points can be perceived in Aquinas's own work.

Early Christian thinkers critically influenced the presumption of sinfulness that surrounded sex throughout the Middle Ages. Before Aquinas, Saint Augustine's writings in the fifth century were perhaps the most influential in propagating the opinion that sex should solely be performed for the purpose of procreation. Vardy went as far as to say that "Augustine was responsible for turning a generally negative attitude to sex which arose from a desire to maintain the identity of the growing Christian Church in a hostile environment into a negative attitude based on theological principles."

In Augustine's view, sex was a necessary evil that needed to be tolerated with a stiff upper lip and an aura of servitude. Enjoying sex, even within the marital bed, was a sin. When it came time for a married couple to do their duty by God and procreate, they should "descend with a certain sadness" to their unfortunate task. The act was to be performed in this melancholy attitude. This was the only version of sex that was without sin: two long-faced, Tim Burton–esque characters rubbing together with only the hope of a child in mind. If a married couple were motivated to boink solely for the pleasure of boinking, this made them no better than adulterers.

Shall we welcome Augustine himself? Come join us, you naughty boy!

Augustine was no saint when it came to the pleasures of the flesh. Before the age of thirty-two, he was living up the libertine lifestyle. He writes in his *Confessions* (397–400 CE) that by the age of sixteen, he had surrendered himself entirely to the powers of lust:

> *In that sixteenth year of the age of my flesh, when the madness of lust (to which human shamelessness giveth free license, though unlicensed by Thy laws) took the rule over me, and I resigned myself wholly to it.*

Describing himself as "boiled over in [his] fornications," Augustine admitted that sex became his obsession for the first three decades of his life. By seventeen, he had taken a lover, with whom he would remain (if not entirely faithfully) for fifteen years. She would give birth to their son before he dropped her for a ten-year-old heiress. As this child was two years too young for Augustine to marry, he decided to take in another concubine while he waited. As he infamously wrote at the time: "Grant me chastity and continence, only not yet."

I hope it goes without saying that it is only because he was a man that Augustine could act the way he did and still succeed in becoming a Christian saint whose writing profoundly influenced the sexual intolerance of Christian churches to this day. I doubt contemporaries were as forgiving of any of the teenage (and younger) girls involved.

I don't tell you of Augustine's indiscretions in order to condemn him—who am I to condemn a saint?—but I do believe that this kind of information provides vital context about the shaky ground upon which our most stubborn stigmas stand. This contradictory mess is the foundation upon which we have built our ideas of sexual ethics to this very day. It has not only affected our thinking about sexual acts—which, if performed solely for pleasure, are inevitably colored by sinfulness or shame—but also heavily stigmatized attitudes toward contraception. If sex for non-reproductive purposes is bad, then devices designed to prevent this outcome can be nothing other than evil. Followers of Augustine were the first to unequivocally condemn the use of contraception, even between married people. While this marks an important turning point in history, it should also serve as a reminder that methods of sexual protection and contraception existed long before the common era (a point to which we will return).

Over this course, we're going to look at various deviations from the Christian norm of "innocent," procreative sex. We will look through the menu of sexual acts—delights such as oral and rimming—along with the history of contraception itself. We'll wash this down by examining how more liberal attitudes toward relationship structures further challenge the idea that "good" sex takes place only when you're monogamously married and wanting kids.

I promised you this conversation would be wide-ranging and eclectic. I promised you a smorgasbord, too, so let's ease in with something vanilla before moving on to the flavors that might be more of an . . . acquired taste.

By the end of this section, we'll have well and truly tried to unravel what I call the "sin kink": the formative idea of sex as sinful, which continues to centrally influence our thinking around sexual desires and behaviors, even if the most sexually liberated among us don't realize it does. By exploring all these contradictions in the sin kink, we'll ask: Have we fully undone the work of shame as an enduring cultural force attached to sex—thanks to our friends Aquinas and Augustine—or do we still have a long, long way to go?

An Oral History

L et's start with an odd opening gambit. Did you hear that sex is going out of fashion? It's a fact that would perhaps bring Augustine joy: people are refusing to partake in the horizontal tango at the same rate they used to. Imagine, in this sex-crazed society—when degenerate people even feel the need to make history sexy by marketing it as "kinky"—rates of intercourse are actually declining. At a time when we are ostensibly talking about sex more than ever, it seems we are losing interest in putting these words into action.

From the USA to the UK, Germany to Japan, national studies show a decline in partnered sexual activity. The United States saw a significant fall between 2009 and 2018: the percentage of respondents performing penile–vaginal intercourse dropped from 76.5 percent to 71.9 percent; anal intercourse from 20 percent to 17.8 percent; oral sex from 65.3 percent to 60.4 percent; and even acts of mutual masturbation fell from 42 percent to 33.8 percent. Blame cannot even be placed on the dwindling libidos of the older generations, as the most drastic decrease was among adolescents aged fourteen to seventeen: this group saw a striking 50 percent cutback in all partnered sexual activity.

We are losing the desire to place swords in sheaths—and, what's more, professionals are becoming increasingly anxious:

Researchers have expressed concern about such declines, given the conse-
quences on human fertility and relationship happiness as well as what poten-

tial declines in partnered sexual frequency may reflect about the influences of social media platforms, environmental influences on people's hormones, and overall changes to human connection and intimacy.

Long gone are the days of moral panic surrounding the prevalence of sex, drugs, and rock and roll; authorities are now encouraging people to get back to doing the no-pants dance.

One UK study, which noted that the "frequency of sex has declined recently in Britain," also listed the numerous health benefits that have been associated with sex.

Research indicates that men and women who enjoy an active sex life are fitter, happier, and have better cognitive function and increased life expectancy. Evidence shows that sexual activity might help prevent infection by bolstering immune function; protect against cardiovascular disease by lowering heart rate and blood pressure; and reduce stress by increasing release of oxytocin.

The doctor's orders? Sex *at least* once a week: "The UK NHS [National Health Service] considers the evidence to be sufficiently convincing to recommend sexual activity for its health enhancing effects, with the claim, 'Weekly sex might help fend off illness.'" I will take that over an apple a day, any day.

Alternative studies suggest that not all sexual activities are in decline; it is just vaginal sex that is losing its slippery hold on the public. Indeed, by virtue of popularity, oral activities could be the new contender for prom queen.

When comparing the results from Australia's national survey from 2001 to 2012, one of the most statistically significant increases to be found is the rate of people who were having oral sex. By 2012, 80 percent of women reported engaging in oral sex at some stage in their lifetime, an increase of 15 percent from the previous decade. (No one goes down under better than us Down Under.) Even in our own survey conducted for this book, oral sex was more popular than vaginal sex, with 86.3 percent of participants enjoying an "Australian kiss" in the previous year, versus 81.8 percent doing it the P-in-V way.

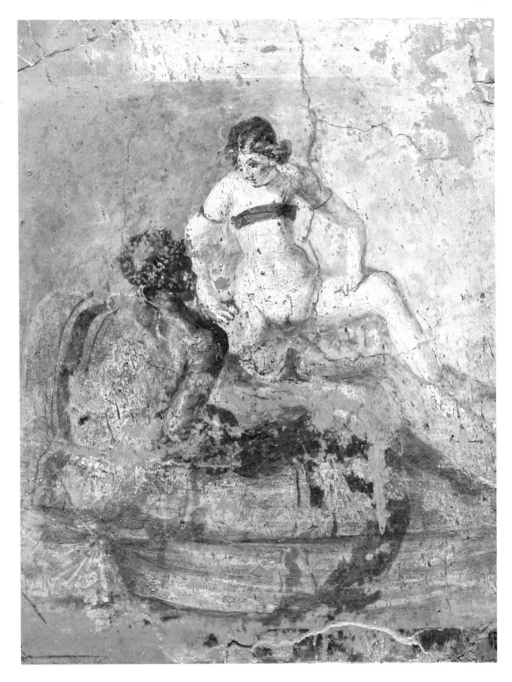

This fresco, currently in the collection of the Secret Museum in Naples, portrays an enticing erotic scene in ancient Pompeii, dating to the first century CE.

This is where language presents a problem. All the national studies declaring SEX IS ON THE DECLINE were referring to only one form of partnered sexual activity—an act between two heterosexual individuals, which, largely, was defined as the placing of a penis into a vagina. It in no way reflected the fact that other forms of sex, such as oral activities, are on the rise. Nor did it reflect the fact that homosexual and other categorically queer encounters are similarly experiencing a spike in popularity. The discrepancy between claims that sex is going out of fashion and the fact that other acts—which many would classify as sex—are on the rise begs yet another, more fundamental question:

What even *is* sex?

Let's start the long answer to that question with a quick oral history.

One of the earliest recorded examples comes from ancient Egyptian mythology. After her brother (who is also her husband) is chopped into pieces, the goddess Isis seeks to restore his life—however, one crucial body part is missing. Isis forges an artificial penis for her brother-husband and gives him (literally) the best oral sex of all time, essentially blowing him back to life.

In surviving ancient Roman brothel sites, artwork depicting the performance of fellatio and cunnilingus can be found along with advertisements for workers who excelled in these services. Erotic pottery remnants from the Moche civilization of ancient Peru depict a variety of heterosexual and homosexual erotic acts—with oral sex far more commonly depicted than the rare celebration of vaginal sex. Meanwhile, in ancient Greece, there were strict etiquette rules around oral sex: it was considered shameful and degrading to perform, while little stigma was attached to the person who received it.

These attitudes, at least in the Western world, were completely turned on their head by Christian thought in the early eighth century. *The Penitential of Theodore* advised confessors how much penance should be dished out as punishment for various sins. By their account, receiving oral sex was even worse than engaging in bestiality: "Someone who sends semen into the mouth shall do penance for seven years: this is the worst of evils." The list of sins progressed from masturbation and sleeping together when unmarried to adultery, bestiality, and anal sex—and then, finally, the act of *receiving* oral sex.

After centuries of being shunned as sinful, oral sex again rears its head in literature from the early modern age. Though it's unlikely to have been pointed out during studies at school, Shakespeare's works are sprinkled with cheeky references to the act. One such reference to the pleasure of "country matters" appears in *Hamlet* (written 1599–1601, published 1604), which is subtle enough for many schoolteachers to quickly skim over.

HAMLET: Lady, shall I lie in your lap?
OPHELIA: No, my lord.
HAMLET: I mean, my head upon your lap?
OPHELIA: Ay, my lord.
HAMLET: Do you think I meant country matters?

A more poetic description is found in Shakespeare's poem *Venus and Adonis* (1593):

Graze on my lips; and if those hills be dry,
Stray lower, where the pleasant fountains lie.

Now, drinking from "pleasant fountains" may sound sexy enough, but is it actually classified as sex?

In 1998, this question would take hold of an entire nation.

"I did not have sexual relations with that woman."

These infamous words would open a wide-ranging conversation on what we consider sex to be. President Bill Clinton and White House intern Monica Lewinsky were involved in the biggest sex scandal the world had ever seen: Clinton was accused of multiple sexual encounters with his much younger subordinate, and denied them all. It later came to light that he had, in fact, received oral sex from Lewinsky. During the deposition, the question was asked: "Have you ever had sexual relations with Monica Lewinsky, as that term is defined in Deposition Exhibit 1?" Clinton reviewed the definition and gave the same answer as he had to the public: "I have never had sexual relations with Monica Lewinsky."

Clinton, in this instance, was recognized to be innocent. Why? Because the act of receiving oral sex was not classified as *sex* as it was defined by the independent counsel's office. As Clinton was to reason in his own words, "I thought the definition included any activity by [me], where [I] was the actor and came in contact with those parts of the bodies . . . with the purpose [or] intent [of] gratification." Clinton had not come into contact with "those parts" of Lewinsky's body during their oral encounter, as she had been the one performing oral on him. By that logic, while Lewinsky was classified as having had sexual relations with him, he had not had sexual relations with her. (He had just pulled down his pants when she happened to be there, I guess.) Clinton was accused of giving a misleading testimony—however, he held strong to his interpretation: that his actions in this encounter did not match the definition of sexual relations.

So, what is sex? In the wake of Sexgate, the *Journal of the American Medical Association* fast-tracked a report by researchers from the Kinsey Institute for Research in Sex, Gender and Reproduction that had asked this exact question. Authors of this 1991 study asked a large sample of male and female university students about the history of their sexual activity and, most important, what they classified as "having sex." The final report was fascinating, exposing the complex and differing definitions of doing the deed. While practically everyone believed that penile–vaginal intercourse classified as sex, a small portion of men (nearly 1 percent) did not even believe that *this* classified. Sadly, no follow-up questions were asked so we can understand exactly what fantastically erotic act these men *would* define as sex.

It could well be that they did not believe that the act of penetration was enough: it is a commonly held belief that ejaculation or orgasm needs to occur in order for sex to have taken place. A similar loophole made headlines in 2021, after a video went viral on TikTok about the practice of "soaking" in the young Mormon community. According to reports, this pastime allowed youthful couples to satisfy their sexual needs while also avoiding the sin and scandal of "having sex." It wasn't just confined to a couple in a bedroom—soaking is basically a threesome. It starts in the same way as many heterosexual encounters, with a penis being inserted into a vagina. This, however, is where our hetero couple must stop. To go any further would be to enter the world of sinful vice and eternal shame. At this point, your handy best friend comes in (not literally):

they are responsible for shaking the bed enough to imitate the motions of thrusting. This way, the couple don't actively have sex—they simply fall onto each other on a shaking bed. While there is no actual evidence of just how common the act of soaking is, it is a well-known rumor at least within the Mormon community, and the since-deleted video discussing it received over a hundred million views on TikTok alone.

To return to our 1991 survey, many other loopholes begin to present themselves. Only 80 percent of people considered anal sex as "having sex"—a definition that may instantly wash away the sins of many people in your life. At the opposite end of the scale, acts that many would consider foreplay are considered by some participants on this survey as going all the way; nearly 14 percent considered touching someone's genitals as sex, 3.4 percent considered touching someone's breasts or nipples as sex, and 2 percent considered deep kissing as sex. That kissing is considered by some to be sex cannot be explained away by the fact that this study took place in ye olde days of the 1990s, when everything was innocent and broadcast in black-and-white, as 3.6 percent of people reported on *our* survey that they considered deep kissing sex. More than half of said people were aged between sixty and seventy-nine, demonstrating the different ideas of sex harbored by the various generations.

How would President Clinton have fared against these definitions? Among these 599 students at Indiana University in 1991, only 40 percent considered oral sex to constitute "amorous congress," so Clinton is again cleared of his charge of sexual relations with that woman—but it's unlikely he would be today, as the parameters of sex continue to shift. In Australia in 2012 to 2013, two thirds (68 percent) of respondents agreed that oral sex constituted having sex. A decade later, in our survey, this number was well in the majority—74.9 percent. Perhaps unsurprisingly, those identifying as LGBTQIA+ were far more likely to consider this as sex; 87 percent of nonbinary and trans men and women were also in agreement with this definition. Cis women (73 percent) were the *least* likely to consider tongue-in-cheek activity as "doing the deed."

Why does it matter that we have such different definitions of sex? These varied understandings have an important impact when trying to understand not only the patterns of sexual behaviors but also our changing attitudes toward them. Researching and understanding sexual behavior becomes complicated when some people classify kissing as intercourse, while others don't even classify penile–vaginal penetration as such.

These discrepancies can give us an understanding of just how easily anything that deviates from the stubbornly held cultural norm of procreative sex can slip through the gaps, even to this day. If oral and anal sex hadn't been included in this study, many queer personalities would not be accounted for in the data. An understanding that *sex* has multiple meanings can go a long way toward helping us discuss and understand contemporary sexuality—and, quite paradoxically, recognizing that its meaning is fluid and malleable seems to be the best way to ensure there is relative consistency in our individual understandings of the topic.

Rimming: Talking in Tongues

N ow let's take a detour through a different kind of oral history, about a sex act that rarely makes it into our textbooks—and that certainly didn't rate a mention from our friends Aquinas and Augustine.

Rimming is the new anal. Rates of anal sex, which used to be so strongly associated with men who have sex with men, are significantly declining. In 2004, 30 percent of homosexual Australian men reported to have received anal penetrative intercourse (the position colloquially known as "the bottom"). However, in the space of a mere decade, that percentage fell to 17, and not because these men began performing anal penetration ("the top"), which followed a similar pattern (falling from 38 percent to 22 percent). Anal has left the building, slamming the back door on its way out. In its place, we find a new ruler—the Tosser of the Salad.

Rimming is on the rise, regardless of gender or sexuality. A new age of ass-kissing has been welcomed in by the younger generation in particular. A recent study found that one in five respondents had received a behind-the-scenes licking in the previous three months. (Although participants thirty-five and above were significantly more likely to have engaged in anal than in rimming.)

While it rarely features in many history documentaries, rimming does have a complex place within the history of sexuality. Put simply, tossing the salad isn't new: *anilingus* was first coined as a term in 1899, in the English translation of Richard von Krafft-Ebing's groundbreaking work, *Psychopathia Sexualis*. It was recognized there as a "perverse" pleasure, a sexual desire to be studied to understand why an individual's interest deviated from the "norm."

Rimming was, of course, practiced for many centuries before we decided to give it a name. Throughout the Middle Ages, it was seen as more comical than anything else. In *The Canterbury Tales* (written 1387–1400), a woman tricks her suitor into confusing one set of cheeks with the other, sending him down to kiss her ass rather than her lips. Rimming was at once everywhere and nowhere. It is rarely mentioned in any written descriptions—and yet, visually, it is omnipresent. The margins of medieval manuscripts were often decorated in beautiful or humorous illustrations, and rimming often made the cut. Depictions of men, monkeys, and dogs (sometimes separately, sometimes all together) licking each other's asses or performing feats of acrobatics to kiss their *own* asses can be found across manuscripts of the time—a fact I discovered on a thread on Twitter (of all places!) by Dr. Erik Wade. While it's a sexual act to us now, these illustrations were jokes—even in medieval times, no one liked a kiss-ass.

There were theological connotations, too. As elucidated by historian Martha Bayless, the backside was associated with filth, and thus sinfulness. It was for this reason that "medieval illustrations of devils often had faces on their groins or backsides, to show that their bodies were as disordered as their morality. Kissing a rear end meant that your morality was distorted."

Indeed, bum-kissing even became associated with witchcraft. To demonstrate their commitment to their master and everything unholy, witches were believed to give the tushy of their horny boss the *osculum infame*, or the "kiss of shame" (a workplace demand that makes sense as their boss was literally Satan), along with writing their names in his special book. Though most often considered as a sign of devotion, some publications from the time suggest it was also believed to be an act of penance. As reported in *Newes from Scotland, Declaring the Damnable Life and Death of Doctor Fian* (1591):

> *And seeing that they tarried over long, hee at their coming enjoyned them all to a pennance, which was, that they should kisse his buttockes, in sign of duety to him, which being put over the pulpit bare, every one did as he had enjoyned them.*

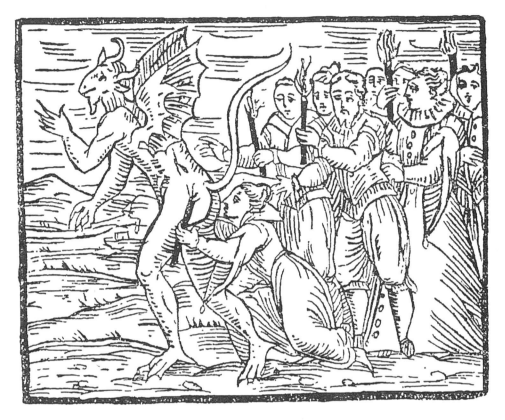

Francesco Maria Guazzo's *Compendium Maleficarum* (1608), a witch-hunter's manual, vividly depicts *osculum infame*, also known as the "kiss of shame."

The cultural significance of rimming was so deeply rooted in sin that indulgence could see you charged with heresy. When the Knights Templar were arrested and charged with heresy on Friday the thirteenth of October, 1307, anal kissing was included in their lists of crimes. The accusations against them bore considerable similarity to those targeted against witches, including suggestions that they were encouraging homosexual practices.

Now, who is that seeking entry to the dining room? What a remarkably small man, very thin and pale, with a profusion of fine, fair hair . . .

Ah, of course! I should have known.

The canonical composer Wolfgang Amadeus Mozart (1756–1791) once wrote a song called "Leck mich im Arsch" (or, in English, "Lick Me in the Arse"). This beautiful canon was written as a party piece, designed to be sung by six voices in a round. After his death, his wife, Constanze Mozart, would send his canons to the publishers—this piece, however, came with a small disclaimer that it may need to be adapted for the sake of propriety. An unadulterated manuscript came to light in 1991. Shall we have a listen?

> Lick my arse!
> Let us be glad!
> Grumbling is in vain!
> Growling, droning is in vain,
> is the true bane of life,
> Droning is in vain,
> Growling, droning is in vain, in vain!
> Thus let us be cheerful and merry, be glad!
> Lick my arse!

This wasn't even his only song to celebrate the joys of ass-licking. Mozart took a canon composed by Wenzel Trnka, originally titled "Nichts labt mich mehr als Wein" ("Nothing Pleases Me More than Wine"), and turned it into a celebration of a far dirtier culinary delight. "Leck mir den Arsch fein recht schön sauber" ("Lick My Arse Right Well and Clean") goes as follows:

> Lick my arse nicely,
> lick it nice and clean,
> nice and clean, lick my arse.
> That's a greasy desire,
> nicely buttered,
> like the licking of roast meat, my daily activity.
> Three will lick more than two,
> come on, just try it,
> and lick, lick, lick.
> Everybody lick their arse for themselves.

Mozart was undoubtedly an ass man. Other writings, such as a series of intimate letters penned to his cousin (and love interest) Maria Anna Thekla Mozart, display an equally passionate fascination with the wonders of the backside. He once tastefully bid her adieu thus:

Well, I wish you good night
But first shit into your bed and make it burst.
Sleep soundly, my love
Into your mouth your arse you'll shove.

Mozart loved scatological humor. In fact, endocrinologist Benjamin Simkin has estimated that thirty-nine of Mozart's letters contained some kind of poo joke. Though bodily and intimate, it is unlikely that these letters were intended to be taken seriously (a phrase such as, "Oui, by the love of my skin, I shit on your nose, so it runs down your chin" isn't exactly a turn-on for most women). Akin to the ass-kissing monkeys and men with faces on their butts that decorated medieval manuscripts, Mozart's poo letters and bum songs were more like dirty inside jokes.

That's not to say, however, that there were no sexual associations with these behaviors. The works of the Marquis de Sade (1740–1814), written around the same period as Mozart's, do not shy away from, well, anything. His pornographic novels, such as *120 Days of Sodom*, are plentiful in their descriptions of characters who have "fondled, kissed, lewdly licked [their] behind, and squirted evidence of [their] virility over [their] cheeks." Indeed, his works celebrate the joys of licking asses for sexual pleasure to the point of obsession. As Sade once wrote, "If it is the dirty element that gives pleasure to the act of lust, then the dirtier it is, the more pleasurable it is bound to be." I shall leave it to your own astute imagination to work out what the "dirty element" is in this context.

A joy to heretics, a source of humor for great composers and writers, and now a sexual practice that is coming well into vogue. According to our survey—which, it must be said, had a sample that was younger and queerer than the general population—one in every four people had experienced oral-anal contact in the previous year.* Indeed, "sinful" licking of all kinds has become a fascination of ours over the past decade, with a whopping total of 89 percent of Melburnians saying they had participated in oral–genital contact in the previous three months.

To summarize: Oral acts of all kinds are up across the board. Anal is up for heterosexual people,† but down for homosexual people. Vaginal sex is significantly down on all accounts.

How can we account for such significant global trends? What causes the popularity of behavior that happens behind closed doors to either plummet or surge?

Studying these trends—from their places in history to the statistics of today—reminds us that our sexual lives are fashioned by a complex interplay of environmental, social, and biological factors. Bum-licking can be a basic part of foreplay or it might have seen you burned at the stake for witchcraft. We have far less control over our fantasies and desires than we would like to believe. What turns us on, what repulses us, what we consider normal, and what we consider inappropriate are far from immutable facts of nature—they are all shaped by the world around us, for better or worse.

---

* In the SexTistics survey, 26.2 percent said they had participated in some form of oral–anal contact in the previous year (Appendix, table 5).

† For heterosexual men in Australia, there was an increase from 21 percent participation in 2004 to 26 percent in 2014. For heterosexual women, there was an increase from 15 percent to 20 percent. There were similar findings in France. See Richard O. de Visser et al., "Change and Stasis in Sexual Health and Relationships: Comparisons between the First and Second Australian Studies of Health and Relationships," *Sexual Health* 11, no. 5 (2014): 505–9, https://doi.org/10.1071/SH14112.

Sense and Syphilis

I t would be impossible to list all the external factors that can affect and have affected our sexual behavior over time. However, I do believe it is worth diverting our attention away from the beautiful songs being performed in the music room (I'm so glad they found six people to sing "Lick Me in the Arse" as a three-part round as intended) to discuss a factor that is often overlooked: access to contraception.

Throughout history, our ability to access contraception—especially safe contraception—has been and remains a critical factor in patterns of sexual decision-making. Far too often, we consider past cultures to have simply placed a high value on "purity," without recognizing the risk of unwanted pregnancies and spread of incurable diseases that they were trying to avoid. By noting behavioral changes around landmark moments—such as the invention of penicillin and the pill—we can see just how greatly access to safety measures can shape the contours of our intimate lives.

Way back in the fourth century, our good friend Aristotle was an advocate for one-child families, as many prominent thinkers of the time were in favor of stabilizing the population to prevent numbers becoming too large to provide for (can you imagine?). Though abortion and infanticide weren't looked upon favorably, they were sometimes *recommended* for the greater good of preventing overpopulation. Yet even in ancient times, prevention was considered the safest policy.

Hippocrates (460–375 BCE)—considered by many as the father of medicine—had some remarkable ideas regarding how to prevent pregnancy. In his work *On the Seed*, he suggests that a woman who "had the habit of going with the men" should "jump up and down, touching her buttocks with her heels at each leap" to evacuate semen following intercourse. Believing obesity would cause infertility, others recommended weight gain to prevent any unwanted pregnancies. The physician Soranus of Ephesus (estimated to have lived between the first and second centuries CE), who wrote a four-volume treatise called *Gynecology*, was also in favor of vigorous movement as a means for anti-conception, with some equally intriguing suggestions.

> *And during the sexual act, at the critical moment of coitus when the man is about to discharge the seed, the woman must hold her breath and draw herself away a little, so that the seed may not be hurled too deep into the cavity of the uterus. And getting up immediately and squatting down, she should induce sneezing and carefully wipe the vagina all round; she might even drink something cold.*

Some approaches bore a little more credibility. Aristotle recommended covering the vagina with cedar oil, a method that finds its roots in ancient Egypt. Other contraceptive methods are listed in what remains of the Kahun Gynaecological Papyrus (1850 BCE)—the oldest medical text in Egypt and the second-oldest text in the entire world—as well as the Ebers Papyrus (1550 BCE), such as inserting a mixture of dates, honey, and gum from acacia leaves into the vagina. A strange method, but one that was likely somewhat successful. When the gum from these leaves is compounded, it essentially becomes spermicide, and is still used in many contraceptive jellies today.

Others, not so much: for example, inserting a soluble block of crocodile feces (mixed with honey) to act as an absorbent sponge for semen. It was also a technique guaranteed to make a lover say, "See you later, alligator," which I suppose makes it an effective contraceptive after all.

Ancient Egyptians may have used early versions of the condom such as linen sheaths, though these were intended to prevent disease more than pregnancy. Even three thousand years ago, people knew that disease could be spread through sexual intercourse, and at the time, Egyptians were concerned about bilharzia, an infection caused by parasitic worms, which could (and does) lead to chronic health issues.

There is some debate regarding whether early condoms can be traced back to ancient times at all, as pregnancy was considered the woman's responsibility, and thus most recorded methods tend to revolve around female contraception. The only male contraceptives recorded reliably are coitus interruptus and coitus per anum—fancy ways of saying "pulling out" and "butt stuff."

With the fall of the Roman Empire, contraceptives declined in popularity. Once the fifth century rolled around, Saint Augustine was there ready to condemn them, while playing absentee father to his out-of-wedlock child. As contraception became stigmatized, awareness of these established methods dwindled. However, the demand (and desire) to prevent pregnancy clearly did not—leading us to turn to increasingly bizarre methods.

Weasels, for whatever reason, took on a starring role in the sex lives of medieval Europeans. In France, it was believed that "if the foot of a female weasel was cut off leaving the animal still alive and the foot dried and hung as a pendant about her neck, the woman would not conceive. If she took it off she would become pregnant immediately." It wasn't just female weasels who got the rough end of the bargain. Toronto's History of Contraception Museum notes, "If one takes the two testicles of a weasel and wraps them up, binding them to the thigh of a woman who wears also a weasel bone on her person, she will no longer conceive." "Pop" *doesn't* go the weasel.

It really takes until the sixteenth century for contraception to regain substantial documentation. This can largely be attributed to the syphilis epidemic that spread through Europe and Asia at the time. This disease did not look like it does today. When it first arrived on the scene, syphilis was far more deadly. As historian Jared Diamond has summarized, "When syphilis was first definitely recorded in Europe in 1495, its pustules often covered the body from the head to the knees, caused flesh to fall from people's faces, and led to death within a few months." It is consequently no wonder that after syphilis arrived in Asia in 1505, recorded uses of condoms simultaneously appear. *Kabuto-gata*, a "helmet" that sits on top of the penis, is recorded in Japan around this time. It was first made of tortoiseshell or horn, though such materials would later be replaced by a thin leather (this was called the *mara-bukuro*, or the "penis-sack").

The first uncontested account of condom use appears around then, used for the purpose of disease prevention rather than contraception, which seems to have been an unexpected bonus rather than its aim. In the sixteenth century, Gabriele Falloppio described the use of linen sheaths that were soaked in a chemical solution before being tied around the penis with a ribbon, like a beautiful little present. Falloppio claimed his invention withheld the trials of scientific experimentation, having tested the preventive device on eleven hundred different men, none of whom contracted syphilis (though all of whom, I imagine, were more than happy to participate in the experiment).

This wasn't the only widespread syphilis epidemic to shake the world. The disease was to rear its head again in the nineteenth century—a fact unlikely to be covered in many Jane Austen adaptations. Regardless, it is an undeniable truth that one in five Londoners had syphilis by the age of thirty-five. If that number isn't shocking enough, the number of Londoners who contracted gonorrhea or chlamydia was far higher. As historian Simon Szreter states:

> *The city had an astonishingly high incidence of STIs at that time. It no longer seems unreasonable to suggest that a majority of those living in London while young adults in this period contracted an STI at some point in their lives.*

Not only was sex already steeped in ideas of sin and shame, now the prevalence of sexually transmitted infections reinforced dominant cultural ideas about sex as dirty—a source of contagion that needed to be controlled.

There was no effective cure found for syphilis (or "the pox") until the beginning of the twentieth century, meaning if you happened to fall within the unlucky 20 percent, there was generally no hope of recovery. Brothels and other forms of sex work, infamously referred to as "the great social evil," were prolific across England during this time. The spread of syphilis and the popularity of these establishments were not entirely unconnected. Admission records of London's hospitals and workhouse infirmaries show that the disease was particularly rife among young, impoverished, mostly unmarried women, who used commercial sex to support themselves. With no effective treatment available, those afflicted were often prescribed mercury (which, thanks to the privileges of science, we know to be just as detrimental as untreated syphilis—if not more so). This led to the popular saying: "A night with Venus, and a lifetime with mercury."

It wasn't only a cure for STIs that was lacking but also preventive methods. While condoms did exist, they were not anywhere near as widely accessible, encouraged, or effective as they are today. One of the major proprietors within Regency London was Mrs. Phillips, who held a shop in Covent Garden. These "condoms designed for gentlemen" were made "of sheep's or goat's gut, pickled, scented, eight inches long, delicately fashioned on glass molds by the hands of the proprietress." While better than nothing, the materials meant these condoms were prone to breaking—and certainly not the sexiest addition to one's affairs. Condoms had become quite widely available during the eighteenth century, sold from pubs and chemists, theaters, and market shops. However, these were readily available only to the middle and upper classes. What made Mrs. Phillips notable is that she primarily catered to female sex workers, servicing the market for which no one else was accounting. She dedicated herself to creating "implements of safety" for her customers, advertising her wares as such:

> *To guard yourself from shame or fear*
> *Votaries to Venus, hasten here*
> *None in our wares er'er found a flaw*
> *Self-preservation's Nature's law.*

It would not be until the 1910s that the first effective treatment for syphilis was developed: the drug Salvarsan. By the 1940s, a safe and accessible cure was established with the production of penicillin—one of two inventions in that decade that would truly change our sex lives forever.

Lord of the Pills

The invention of "the pill" was nothing short of life-changing. My nan speaks about this as the moment she stopped living in fear and started living as an adult woman. It gave women the option, perhaps for the first time, to be active in their sexuality and in control of their own fertility. With the pill in hand, women took control of their professional careers, the decision about (and timing of) becoming a mother, and the size of their family.

Without exaggeration, the pill can be credited for changing the course of history and the shape of a new social identity. What it offered to women was freedom—a freedom that had been enjoyed by their male counterparts from near time immemorial. This freedom is not even a hundred years old.

While the pill was invented in the 1940s by Dr. Carl Djerassi, it would not become commercially available until the 1960s. Even then, however, it was initially available only to married women. The assumption was that "birth control" would, for the respectable married woman, do just that—*control* the timing of birth rather than prevent procreation altogether. However, the demand extended quickly. Statistical studies showed that sexual activity outside marriage had been skyrocketing since the 1940s, and there was a need to prevent the rising number of births taking place outside these sacred bounds. The impact of the world wars almost certainly ushered in this era of sexual revolution and liberation. As remarked by historian Alan Petigny:

After 15 years of Depression and war, there was also a desire on the part of
Americans to live in the moment and enjoy life, and they were accordingly less
likely to defer to traditional restraints on their behavior.

During wartime, gender roles and rules of sexual conduct had undergone a period of obscurity, changing the shape of family life entirely. Women's place was no longer confined to the domestic home, as they became workers and volunteers while their fathers, husbands, and sons were sent on overseas assignments without knowing when they would return.

Concepts of sexual propriety became ever more blurred. While the number of extramarital relationships that took place during this time is largely undocumented, data from symptomatic outcomes can give us an indication. During World War I, it is estimated that seven million man-days of service were lost due to venereal disease. The sheer scope of this spread caused drastic action to be taken to contain it. In 1938, Congress passed the National Venereal Disease Control Act, which "provided funds for local VD clinics and diagnostic equipment to private practitioners." Pamphlets were published and handed out to educate troops on sexual hygiene and safe practices— and most important, millions of men were introduced to the condom. Condoms were distributed to American troops during World War II, just as they had been distributed to British troops in World War I. The mix of education about and access to protective means went a long way in slowing the spread of venereal disease by the end of the war.

Quite ironically, war and disease—two very unsexy things to think about—were accountable for the rising rates of horniness in the early years of the twentieth century. At the start of the 1920s, 86 percent of women reported that they had never slept with anyone before marriage—but by the end of the decade, this number had decreased to 61 percent. Alfred Kinsey, the prolific biologist and sexologist behind this report, claimed that these figures could be directly related to one phenomenon taking America by storm: "cuddle parties." Also known as petting parties, these get-togethers became popular in the 1920s following the devastation of the 1918 influenza pandemic. Coming out of a period of war and isolation, people felt touch-starved and in need of human connection—a feeling to which I am sure many of us can relate.

Cuddle parties were exactly what they sound like: with your chosen partner for the night, you would explore physical contact through hugging. One survey at the time estimated up to 92 percent of all college students were participating in them. They were praised as a new way to test intimacy before marriage, while also alleviating that anxiety surrounding human touch caused by the pandemic. However, this wholesome joy couldn't last forever. Cuddle parties were eventually banned in some places, with fears that all that hugging may lead to something more. Some couples were even fined at these events for taking things a little too far when their hugs progressed into spooning (*the scandal!*).

Medical advancements in contraceptive methods and disease prevention have revolutionized our sex lives over the past century—but, as we will see, this is not a straightforward tale of ever-increasing freedom. History is always there to complicate the stories we tell ourselves.

I believe it is time for our plates to be cleared. How have you enjoyed your aperitives?

Now, come. Let us gather around the piano while we wait for the next course to be served. Mozart has found a brave singer; I've never heard the "Queen of the Night" aria performed with quite so many fart noises before. Let us join them, and let us be glad!

At this stage in the evening, we must retrench. We've dived into specific detail about a range of sexual acts, and it's been a great deal to digest. It's plain to see that our sexual behavior is a complex and continual interplay of the unique environmental and biological factors that impact each person's life differently. Looking to how sex lives of the past were influenced might provide insight into how we are affected today. But these are discussions that deserve a dinner course of their own.

Before we get there, let's explore another dimension of the sin kink.

Living in Sin

My dearest Victor, you are here at last. Oh, my apologies: I'm not sure if you have met?

This is Victor Hugo (1802–1885). You are, perhaps, familiar with his works, such as *The Hunchback of Notre-Dame* and *Les Misérables*? I believe it is best to judge the quality of an author by the number of musical adaptations to their name. Give it a few hours and Hugo will be gathering us round the piano for a chorus of "Do You Hear the People Sing?"

You can always trust that a dinner party will become quite rowdy when Hugo is around. That is, when he finds time to attend. See, Hugo is a far more prolific host than I am. It's believed that for much of his life, he would have at least thirty dinner guests at his house every night—many of whom he entertained with his vanishing-orange party trick, in which he would fit an orange and many sugar cubes into his mouth, washing the chewed-up mass down with kirsch. Comforter, philosopher, bon viveur, to be sure.

Hugo was no stranger to biting off more than he could chew. Between writing best-selling novels, getting himself exiled from his home country, and inviting dozens of people to his house every single night, he also found time to become one of the horni-est people in recorded history. He boasted in his diaries that on his wedding night he had copulated with his wife, Adele Foucher, at least nine times. Foucher was far from impressed with her new husband's insatiable libido, and though she managed five pregnancies within eight years, she would call quits on their love life after the youngest child was born.

Hugo and Foucher's situation was not too dissimilar from one that many married couples find themselves in today. Indeed, it seems that marriage is the ultimate cock-block. Across studies, frequency of sex declines with couples who are married. While this could well be due to the natural calming of passion that takes place in a long-term relationship, that cannot explain why rates continue to remain high for people who are cohabiting, rather than married. Statistically, living with someone leads to more sex. Cohabiting women between the ages of sixteen and forty-four reported a median frequency of six sexual encounters a month, married women said four, and divorced or separated said one, while the average single woman said she had not had sex in the past few weeks. Some strange magic takes place after the exchange of rings that significantly decreases the rate of special adult hugs. Wedded sex may be less sinful in the eyes of the Church, but it also happens less often.

Hugo, however, was not overly fazed by Adele's decision (or about her subsequent love affair with his friend Sainte-Beuve). He was off to conquer the rest of Paris—a fact we know because, along with his high libido, Hugo also had a compulsive need to write everything down. Anticipating these nosy historians of the future who feel the need to recount and publicize the sex lives of famous figures (*Deplorable! What has academia come to?*), Hugo used coded language when recording his sexual encounters. When he wrote about a woman's *suisses* (meaning "Swiss"), he was referring to her breasts—an analogy he made because Switzerland was renowned for its milk. Similarly, when he wrote about *poële* (meaning "stove"), he was referring to pubic hair—because *poële* was a homophone for *poil* (meaning "pubic hair"). Once the code was cracked, we were left with a pretty good idea of what his sex timetable looked like.

> *It was not unusual for him to make love to a young prostitute in the morning, an appreciative actress before lunch, a compliant courtesan as an aperitif, and then join the also indefatigable Juliette for a night of sex.*

Perhaps I should look at Hugo's menu for inspiration for future parties?

Hugo was such a large part of the Parisian nightlife that on the day he died, every single brothel in Paris closed for a day of mourning. Workers and friends were given the time to pay their respects to their loyal client. One police officer even reported that sex workers around the city draped their genitals in black crepe as a sign of respect. Urban legend has it that his funeral turned into one of the biggest parties of the year, and there was a baby boom in Paris nine months later. He would have been proud.

Relationships today, of course, look very different than in Hugo's day. Prior to marriage or any form of long-term commitment, contemporary couples are far more likely to test out their sexual compatibility (the try-before-you-buy method). This allows for any discrepancies in libido to be brought to light before or while the bounds of the relationship are negotiated. Perhaps these days Hugo would not have opted for marriage at all. It is easy to see him fitting in well in the age of casual hookups and dating apps.

While apps seem to dominate the world of love, sex, and relationships today, it is strange to think that this era of digital courtship is only ten years old. What a wonderful decade it has been, filled with swiping right, mulling over the perfect bio, and posing proudly with dead fish. In 2022, 4.5 million Australians used dating apps, making it the most common way to find a partner. Around a quarter stated they were using these platforms to find a long-term partner, with the largest demographic of users aged twenty-five to thirty-four. Long gone are the days of casually meeting in a pub or feeling a spark across the room—dating is now a matter of carefully selected profile pictures and setting your preferred radius.

We have a tendency to mourn ye olde days of rom-com-style romance, regarding apps as a colder strategy. Swiping through profiles and forming judgments within a couple of seconds can, understandably, feel a little extreme. But for many users there has been a trade-off: a newfound sense of control and empowerment. Romance is no longer left in the hands of fate and convenience. It does not depend upon meeting your soul mate in high school (a fact that is, statistically, very unlikely), or bumping into them at the bookstore you happen to frequent. Dating apps have opened us up to worlds of romantic possibilities outside our personal bubbles.

I met my partner online at the start of 2020, only a matter of weeks before the world as we knew it turned topsy-turvy. If it hadn't been for the apps, we wouldn't have met at all. It's really as simple as that. We had no mutual friends, we worked in dissimilar fields, and he would much rather have been kicking a soccer ball around while I attended the theater. There is no way our circles would have ever collided—a fact that fills me with as much dread as it does gratitude.

Two and a half years after I swiped onto his profile, we were in the process of unpacking the boxes of our first house together.

Beyond locational convenience or a timely meeting, our observations of each other's profiles and our messaging interactions revealed a shared sense of humor, compatible priorities of family and career, and two ambitious and caring personalities. A quick drink after a day of messaging confirmed all those deductions. We never looked back. In a matter of two weeks, we went from strangers to a team that would support each other through the steep ups and downs of Melbourne's lockdowns.

One of the great advantages of meeting via a dating app is that it was clear from the beginning what each of us was looking for. There wasn't any confusion that he was looking for a long-term relationship while I wanted a quick hookup. Our intentions were shared. It is hard to casually broach such topics in real life. Asking someone you've just met at a club if they're also looking for someone to settle down with is likely to be an awkward conversation, to say the least. A simple check mark on your profile renders that awkwardness obsolete.

This feature has, for some women, been an empowering development. Even in a post–*Sex and the City* world, casual hookups for women remain heavily stigmatized. Dating apps have gone part of the way toward changing this: the very ability to select what you are interested in—be it a no-strings-attached hookup, an ongoing friends-with-benefits situationship, or something a little more "serious"—has granted a lot of women permission to even consider this range of possibilities for themselves. The ability to say you are currently looking for sex and nothing more has truly changed the game when it comes to taking control of our love lives and sexuality. (*Perish the thought!* says our prudish friend Aquinas.) This openness can also allow us to have more honest conversations with potential partners, which in turn can lead to more ethical and respectful relationships, whether casual or long term.

We cannot ignore that there are potential pitfalls, too. Since the emergence of the apps, debate has publicly raged over user safety. Of course, the possibility of stalking or being lied to and manipulated were dangers that existed in the dating world long before it went virtual. If anything, dating apps have only highlighted the existence of these issues within relationships way before Tinder came on the scene.

The growing acceptance of hookup culture and dating apps has generated important, widespread conversation about how to stay safe in our romantic endeavors. Dating will never be the same, which opens a whole new world of risks and possibilities.

Love and Friends
(with Benefits)

Relationships, and how we structure them, are comparably different today from even five years ago—let alone how they were in nineteenth-century Paris, or indeed when Aquinas and, long before him, Augustine were formulating their morality codes about sex and sin. What has for millennia been condemned as "deviant" behavior—premarital sex, one-night stands, casual hookups, open relationships, polyamory; that is, situations in which sex is pursued more for pleasure than for procreation—is being destigmatized by cultural and technological change. Just as we are constantly altering our views of what constitutes sex and what should be labeled as sinful, we are shifting the goalposts around the relationship structures that shape our sexual behavior.

These conversations surrounding love, romance, and sexuality have brought with them an increasing awareness of alternative dynamics, such as open relationships and/or polyamory—whether we have heard about them, known a friend who has tried them, or partaken ourselves. This cultural shift has also coincided with the rising awareness of one crucial statistic: the rates of divorce.

*Half of all marriages end in divorce.**

* While this statistic has been commonly quoted since the 1980s, it has since been debunked. Divorce rates have actually dropped, but so have marriage rates, especially with millennials. See, for example: Belinda Luscombe, "The Divorce Rate Is Dropping. That May Not Actually Be Good News," *Time*, November 26, 2018.

This number was a game changer across the generational divide. For my parents' generation, it came as almost a comfort blanket: a sign it was OK to do what they'd for so long wanted to do. For my generation, it came as a slap in the face. What good were all those Disney films if the prince was going to fuck off when the going got tough? That figure heralded the end of the happily-ever-after (or, at the very least, confirmed its inevitable demise). The illusion was broken, priorities began changing. Our vision began to become more focused, clearer; it wasn't so much the growing old we were fantasizing about, but the here and now (and the soon to be). I've never been averse to pain, but for that slap, I'm particularly grateful.

Death of the family! of the sanctity of marriage! a chorus of conservatives cries.

For those people, I happily display our rates of birth, marriage, and other declared relationships. We are still doing families—we are just doing them differently.

And by differently, as always, I mean more in line with the existence of arrangements other than the nuclear family since the dawn of time. Polyamory and open relationships date back to the ancient world, though often without prioritizing the ethics and consent embedded in these relationship structures today.

In particular, polygamy (the practice of being in multiple marriages at once) appears often in the historical record, and was common for the male partner. In ancient Greece, it was standard for men to have multiple wives and concubines, as well as male lovers. This was especially true for the upper classes. In fact, it was considered a sign of great wealth and status. Homosexual relationships were accepted and celebrated, with the "ideal" of pederasty involving an older man mentoring and having a sexual relationship with a younger man—a topic we will come back to over our next course.

While not as common as it was in Greece, polygamy was practiced by men of higher status in Rome. Concubinage—in which a man could keep a secondary wife who was not entitled to the same legal rights as the primary wife—was also common, particularly among couples who came from different social classes (as a way of evening out the power imbalance). Taking multiple wives was also an ordinary story among the higher classes of ancient Egypt, Mesopotamia, and China, especially by the emperors of the time.

There are also a number of indigenous cultures that have traditionally practiced some form of polyamory or polygamy. The Mosuo people of China have something called "walking marriage," in which women are free to take multiple partners at once and change these partners at will. The Himba people of Namibia practice a similar form of polygamy called "fraternal polyandry," in which brothers share a wife, a practice found in other cultures throughout the world. And on the note of keeping it in the family, the "ghost marriages" of the Nuer people of Sudan allow a man to marry the wife of his brother as a stand-in if the brother happens to pass away. Any children conceived thereafter would be considered as belonging to the deceased husband. And you thought Hamlet was haunted by the ghosts of his past.

Examples of polyamorous communities extend well into the nineteenth century, particularly in religious communities. In fact, that's where we get the term "free love." The Oneida Community was founded in upstate New York in 1848 by John Humphrey Noyes, who is credited with coining the phrase. This perfectionist religious community practiced "complex marriage," in which sex was allowed and encouraged between consenting adults:

> Complex marriage meant that everyone in the community was married to everyone else. All men and women were expected to have sexual relations and did. The basis for complex marriage was [that] the Pauline passage about there being no marriage in heaven meant that there should be no marriage on earth, but that no marriage did not mean no sex.

They also believed in the idea of "male continence," in which men avoided orgasm during sex, as a means of contraception (I can hear Augustine rolling in his grave). Sex, denied the purpose of reproduction, served its own social purpose, allowing "the sexes to communicate and express affection for one another." The community had a complex system of sexual relationships and rules, and it was in operation for over thirty years.

This rich heritage of alternative relationship structures—along with rising divorce rates—have led many academics to question whether humans are naturally monogamous at all. American psychologist David M. Buss has argued that humans, especially men, are biologically inclined toward nonmonogamy, stating that studies point to 40 to 50 percent of men engaging in extramarital relationships at some stage. (For women, the number is 20 to 30 percent.) Sexual variety is one of the primary motivators of infidelity for men—when the opportunity to have sex arises, it seems illogical to say no. Marital happiness generally has little to do with their decision to cheat, whereas low marital satisfaction is the primary reason women do. For women, it's less about presented opportunity and more about having a backup mate in case the first one doesn't work out.

Despite many research papers and projects on the topic, there is still no consensus on whether humans are naturally monogamous, polygamous, or just plain horny. To make matters more difficult, studies into our "natural" inclinations also must keep up with our rapidly changing social situations. Are women naturally more predisposed to monogamy than men, or has their historical oppression led to a dependence on the household provider? What will the future look like now that it is more possible for parents to raise children alone while also earning a living? Changes in gender roles and expectations will ripple and have rippled into the world of romance. How are we meant to navigate new partnerships along such uncertain shores?

Luckily, some academics have come up with theories on how to predict whether a relationship will last—theories that look instead to non-biological factors. Psychologist John Gottman has claimed he is able to predict which newlyweds will get divorced with 90 percent accuracy. The signs are predictable. It all comes down to negative communication patterns—did conflict discussion begin with "harsh start-ups" such as criticism, contempt, or defensiveness? If these communication patterns are left unchecked, Gottman believes they are certain indicators that a relationship breakdown is in store.

This logic can be applied to all relationship structures. Perhaps our increasing exposure to alternative dynamics—which characteristically, although not always, prioritize honest communication—could be why we're seeing positive changes in how we communicate with our partners.

For one thing, cheating is going out of fashion. Recent data shows we are less tolerant than ever of partners having sex outside of a committed relationship. In 2004, 77 percent of men and women believed that this transgression was always wrong. By

2014, these numbers had risen respectively to 85 percent and 82 percent. While we don't have the data yet, I would wager that that number has continued to rise as the past decade has played out.

But why? If we've all been slapped in the face by the divorce statistic (some enjoying that slap far more than others) and we're all disillusioned by the institution of marriage, then wouldn't we expect to be *more* accepting of extramarital relations? It comes down to how we have decided to define one term: *committed relationship*.

In the past decade, Google searches for words related to polyamory and open relationships increased significantly. It used to be rare to hear discussion of alternative relationship structures, and a desire for monogamy was generally just assumed. In the previous study the very large majority of people (96 percent) expected they and their partner would not have sex with anyone else. Yet only 48 percent of men and only 64 percent of women said they had discussed this expectation and agreed upon it with their partner. I believe that one of the reasons we're far less OK with cheating today is because we've opened a space to converse and negotiate what you want out of a relationship—and what you want outside of it. Cheating is going to be a widespread problem when people are trapped into thinking that monogamy is the only way. Equally, cheating becomes far less excusable when there is a plethora of other options, and opportunities for discussion, that can be negotiated with the other party or parties.

This change in information doesn't lie just in shifting cultural attitudes but also with researchers and how we research. It's fair to say that in conducting many of these studies, researchers have often equated romantic love (and security) with sexual exclusivity. Being confronted by your own data telling an entirely different story can be a breakthrough that many would rather ignore. While the minority of people in conducted studies engage in consensual nonmonogamy,* this group reported comparatively high levels of satisfaction. And the reasons aren't too surprising. Healthy consensually nonmonogamous (CNM) relationships hinge upon two things: trust and

---

* For example, in the 2012 national US survey of people in a relationship, 89 percent were monogamous, 4 percent were in open relationships, and 8 percent reported nonconsensual nonmonogamy (i.e., cheating). (See Ethan Czuy Levine et al., "Open Relationships, Nonconsensual Nonmonogamy, and Monogamy among US Adults: Findings from the 2012 National Survey of Sexual Health and Behavior," *Archives of Sexual Behavior* 47, no. 5 (July 2018): 1439–50, https://www.doi.org/10.1007/s10508-018-1178-7.)

communication. While these are ostensibly important factors for any relationship, for a CNM structure to work (or, indeed, be established) at all, detailed conversation needs to take place about the wants, boundaries, and desires of all parties: a conversation that is continued as situations and people change over time. The functioning of this dynamic then relies on the trust each party has that their boundaries are respected.

It is unsurprising, then, that people who have negotiated a CNM relationship report high levels of satisfaction and trust and low levels of jealousy. They are continually employing the two central tenets upon which any healthy relationship dynamic must operate: trust and communication. Imagine if we were to bring this openness into all our relationships. We can do far greater justice to our status as individuals—with our quirks, desires, and fantasies—than we do by stamping the same, one-size-fits-all label on every relationship. Imagine how much frustration, anger, and jealousy could be dissolved by the presence of a recurring simple question—What do *you* want?—and the chance to answer it honestly.

One stubborn stigma holds that a person is interested in open relationships only if they are unsatisfied with their primary partner. Yet studies have found just the opposite. Indeed, one has stated that relational well-being had more influence on people's sexual choices than relationship structure did: "When people feel in control of their sexual encounters and are engaging in sex because they value sex or want to experience pleasure and closeness, they are likely to feel more fulfilled and happier in their relationships, regardless of whether they are in a monogamous or CNM partnership."

It does make you wonder how many stories in history would have been different if we'd had an equivalent concept of CNM partnerships back then. Like our friends Foucher and Hugo, for example. With both partners partaking in extramarital affairs—and heated accounts later in their lives indicating that it became a source of tension for them—I wonder if their relationship could have been less strained if it had existed within a structure more suited to both of their desires. We are far from the first people to feel confined by the bounds of lifelong monogamy.

If we are going to sit here discussing theories of monogamy, then there is really one person we should consult. Most honored guest, allow me to introduce to you a most distinguished gentleman. Verily, the visage of him could best be described as that of a mad scientist, albeit one of great renown. His hair, which resembles a bird's nest most peculiarly, defies all attempts at taming. One cannot help but wonder if it were not concealing a veritable laboratory of ideas and inventions. Yet despite his odd appearance, I believe you will find Mr. Einstein to be a most engaging and entertaining dinner companion.

Now, the ideas of Albert Einstein (1879–1955) changed the world of science and philosophy forever—and yet his ideas regarding relationships and love have gone relatively unremarked. It is high time we discussed Einstein's lesser-known philosophy, his theory of infidelity.

Monogamy was not a concept of which Einstein thought too highly. As he once wrote, "When a man forces himself to remain monogamous, it is a bitter fruit for everyone involved." Einstein was married twice, remaining faithful to neither wife. He lived and even conceived a child with his first wife, Mileva Maric, before they married. It is estimated that he slept with at least ten other women over the course of their marriage, before eventually leaving Mileva for one of his mistresses (who also happened to be his first cousin). But Elsa Löwenthal was in for similar luck. Old habits being hard to kill, Einstein was soon playing the same old game. Among the extramarital relationships, he embarked on a passionate affair with his secretary, and even suggested to her that she should come and live with Elsa and him—an offer she refused, leading Einstein to humorously remark that she had more appreciation "for the difficulties of triangular geometry than I."

It was Einstein's unwavering belief that humans were not meant to be monogamous creatures. As he advised a friend in 1915:

> I am sure you know that most men (as well as quite a number of women) are not monogamously endowed by nature. . . . Nature will come through even stronger if convention and circumstances are putting resistances in the way of the individual.

This theory was heavily one-sided. While he believed men should and would enjoy any number of affairs, wives were expected to passively accept the infidelity: "You should be able to respond to his sins with a smile, and not make a case of war out of it." Indeed, after a brief period of separation from Mileva, Einstein wrote a list of conditions she must accept if they were to continue living together. Among the many demands for chores, cooking, and assistant work, Einstein instructed his wife, "You will not expect any intimacy from me, nor will you reproach me in any way."

The largest problem with Einstein's extramarital affairs is not the affairs themselves—it is the fact that he did not stick to the rule that he'd laid out for himself: "One should do what one enjoys, and won't harm anyone else."

Our detours into the intimate lives of these luminaries expose yet another kink in our thinking. Sure, increasingly liberal models for relationships and hookups can be of huge benefit in destigmatizing our attitudes about sex, and it is wonderful that consent, trust, and communication are evoked more than ever before. But when unequal power dynamics, particularly along the lines of gender, shape those conversations, how "free" can we really say we are?

A Degree of One's Own

.

I t is perhaps unsurprising that Einstein turned out to be such a horny bugger. Education is one of the many unexpected environmental factors that directly correlate with our sexual preferences. The correlation between higher levels of education and people with more liberal attitudes is statistically significant. People who have attained a post–high school degree are twice as likely to engage in masturbation, especially with the use of a bedroom toy (a fact that may explain why theses take quite so long to write).

When academics are not locked away with their research papers and Danny the Dildo, their studies have also found an increase in the number of sexual partners. Having more than ten sexual partners in your lifetime is associated with higher social class and education, while having sex earlier in life is associated with the opposite. If all this isn't enough to encourage you to keep studying, going to university is also associated with homosexuality. Having more education correlates with increased same-sex experience: with less than a high school education, 4 percent of men and 9.7 percent of women reported a same-sex experience; with a post–high school education, these numbers rose to 8.5 percent for men and 13.6 percent for women. Indeed, of those who identified as homosexual on the latest Australian national survey, 65 percent had a post–high school education.

So, it's official—going to university makes you gay.

"Not quite, Esmé." I can hear that frustrated note of disappointment in my mum's voice from across the room. "There is an important difference between *correlation* and *causation.* These studies show a *correlation*; the higher your level of education, the higher your likelihood of identifying with a queer identity and/or engaging in same-sex activities. It doesn't mean, as your *causation* logic would have it, that undertaking a PhD will magically turn you into a lesbian."*

Be that as it may, there is nothing more orgasmically powerful than a woman with multiple degrees. Across these studies, women in general consistently had significantly higher scores on the scale of sexual liberalism than men (p < 0:001, i.e., "statistically significant"). The most advanced technology in the world is perhaps not equipped to record the liberalism of a woman with high levels of education. It seems letting us into their universities was a good idea after all.

In fact, if you want to be certain about . . . finishing, then statistically, you should sleep with a woman. One study collected data from both homosexual and heterosexual men and women—in both cases, the percentage of people who had orgasms during their most recent sexual encounters was greater if they had done it with a woman. Nearly 80 percent of women climaxed when with another woman, compared with only 66 percent when with a man, irrespective of how they sexually identified. Women are far more likely to achieve climax if a range of activities is incorporated into a sexual encounter, rather than being limited to a singular act of stock-standard penetration; indeed, women have been found to orgasm 90 percent of the time when a mixture of oral stimulation and anal/vaginal penetration is performed. Perhaps women are just more attuned to one another's bodily needs. That said, it's not just other women who benefit from these womanly graces. Heterosexual men were more likely to climax than homosexual men, 92 percent compared with 76 percent. So basically, if you want a job done well (or, in some cases, done at all), then you should entrust it to a woman.

It is then surprising that, consistently across studies of opposite-sex partners, far greater numbers of sexual partners are reported for men—twice as many, in fact. This is a statement shared around so many dinner tables and Facebook comment sections that it has almost become gospel. This commonly wielded statistic has some merit: in the national surveys from Australia, the US, and the UK, men reported having more sexual partners than women. In many cases, the number *is* almost double. In a study

---

* An actual conversation I had with my mum after I said this one silly thing during the research process.

of the UK population between 2010 and 2012, men reported an average of 14.1 partners, while women reported 7.1. In a study of the Australian population at the same time, men similarly had an average of 17.7 partners compared with 8.4 for women.

And yet this fact does not stand up to a second of scrutiny.

There are roughly the same number of men in this world as there are women. Let's imagine there are two teams, as the media would often have us believe. It should then be possible that each person from Team Man can choose two players from the other team to make contact with, while Team Woman may each choose only one man to make contact with. The result is an utter mind-fuck, and mathematically impossible. And yet, studies will continue to find that men report having had sex with eighteen women throughout their life, and women will report having had sex with eight men.*

The most interesting insight from these studies is not the number of sexual partners reported, but the cultural and social factors that play a role in the discrepancies. The most obvious explanation would be that men tend to exaggerate their sexual endeavors while women play theirs down—a variable referred to as a "social desirability bias." These gendered expectations will come as no surprise—there is a stubbornly persisting stigma that having many sexual partners makes a woman an undesirable "whore," while the same number would make a man a "hero."

There is some sign of this gap closing. In our survey, the average number of partners for males was 16.3 and for females was 12.2. However, to see the immense influence this cultural myth still holds, consider one particular study.

An experiment was conducted in the US to see just how results were being skewed in self-reports of sexual experience. Participants were split into three groups to answer questions about their histories: group one answered the anonymous questions in a private room; group two were convinced that their answers could be seen by a supervisor; and group three were hooked up to a (fake) lie detector.

Group two, as expected, answered the lowest, with a reported average of 2.6 sexual partners. Group one was slightly higher, with an average of 3.4. It was group three— hooked up to the detector—who answered the highest, with a reported average of 4.4.

---

* While this data relates to the reported experiences of heterosexual and bisexual people, LGBTQIA+ answers don't substantially affect these rates due to significantly smaller numbers.

When the pressure of a lie detector was added, the average number of sexual partners reported by women became practically identical to the number reported by men. Men who completed this study had a similar pattern of results to the women, though their figures were nowhere near as drastically varied.

Women are also far more likely to have had experiences they would forgo reporting, because they regretted them or because they were traumatic. There are also many demographics who are generally not represented in these kinds of studies. Sex workers are often not included as participants in studies about sexual behavior, and women, particularly younger women, make up the majority of members of this profession. With regard to the UK national survey, one person stated: "As far as we know, we did not get any prostitutes: one interviewer in the first survey did get to a brothel but they didn't answer." This factor would certainly skew results, particularly as men are the primary customers of sex workers. If men are reporting these interactions while sex workers are excluded from answering, it's easy to see how yet another discrepancy occurs.

Similarly, reports from the LGBTQIA+ community are regularly disregarded in large-scale studies. Results would likely look a lot different if studies became more inclusive, because statistically speaking, queer people have far more sex than others. When asked to report the number of opposite-sex partners in their lifetime, cis women and cis men reported an average of 12.3 and 18.4 respectively in our survey. Compare those numbers to the prodigious averages of 69.2 opposite-sex partners reported by trans women and 65.1 same-sex partners reported by homosexual men. Queer people have more sex, with more people, than the straights—a fact that, once again, demonstrates the immense influence that social and environmental factors have on our behavior.

This, of course, does not mean *all* queer people are boinking all the time; it merely indicates a culture of liberality that defines some of the queer community. One recent survey noted: "Gay and bisexual men report higher sexual partner numbers, much longer periods of acquiring new partners throughout their lifetime and are more likely to have concurrent sexual partnerships than heterosexual people." It has less to do with sexuality and more to do with the liberality of relationship structures and ideas of sexual relations that characterize the LGBTQIA+ community. "Open relationships" and "friends with benefits" had been features of queer life long before they were adopted by the mainstream, and it is not just these dynamics that have found their way into the wider world—a similar story can be found in some sexual behaviors.

Just as we've redefined what actually counts as sex, and recast our views on what sex is bad, sinful, or deviant, we're also experiencing immense change in our attitudes about how and when we get it on. This flexibility and openness are allowing us to undo enduring cultural hang-ups around equating sex with sin, and looking at the long histories of different behaviors outside the procreative norm allows us to further reduce that stigma. In the words of Lizzo, it's about damn time.

And yet: those cultural hang-ups are a tangled knot, the product of centuries of religion and patriarchy. The project of unpicking that knot will take more than one conversation around the dinner table. Discussions about consent and women's safety are still underway. Discrimination against sex workers continues unabated. LGBTQIA+ people are, in many ways, yet to get a look-in when it comes to our mainstream understanding of sex. Ethical negotiation of alternative relationship structures is of increasing interest, but not everyone is captivated by that conversation.

How far have we come, and how far do we still have to go?

We're freer than ever before. Aren't we?

Ah, there is the bell sounding from the kitchen. Come, let us gather everyone in the dining room. It is time to eat.

THE PLEASURE KINK

Flicking the bean, jerkin' the gherkin, polishing the peanut, cuffing the carrot. What a fine list of foods we have for tonight!

Eat, wank, sleep, repeat. This has been a fine motto since time immemorial. It is an activity in which many of us regularly partake, and yet a topic rarely broached around the dinner table. (Unless, of course, you find yourself sitting at this one.) It sometimes feels as though we only discovered and accepted self-gratification recently, the sex-positive revolution of the 1960s and '70s having gone a long way toward educating us in the various practices and techniques. However, there was a time in human history—it would go without exaggeration to say for the majority of human history—when these little acts of me-time were considered no more scandalous than eating or shitting. In fact, "taking yourself for a walk" was considered such a normal bodily function it rarely receives much attention in depictions or references—and when it does, it is almost always without any sexualization as we would understand it. The term *masturbation* only appears in our vocabulary around the eighteenth century as a result of our sudden desire to *criminalize* the act. Until this time, we were doing it like monkeys—who, along with many other animal species, have been found to enact the words of the Divinyls' hit single.

But why do we masturbate? Is it an inadequate substitute for partnered sex? The stats tell a different story. Far from the prevailing stigma as an activity for the lonely, the more sexual partners you have, the more likely you are to enjoy the five-finger shuffle. Let's just look at this one finding: men who had had *no* sexual partners in a year were 69 percent (nice) likely to have masturbated, whereas men who had had two or more partners were 91 percent likely to have enjoyed this pastime. That is a pretty sizable increase!

Rather than an activity to simply fill the void, masturbation goes a long way toward helping to increase our libido. Quite ironically, one of the signs of a healthy, burgeoning relationship is often thought to be an increase in acts of self-pleasure, as both parties experience a peak in hormonal fires. This is not too dissimilar to the social role masturbation is believed to have played in ancient Greece, where it was considered a healthy substitute for other sexual pleasures. Engagement in self-enjoyment was thought to protect against the destructive force of sexual frustration and thus curb the rates of adultery, which was considered extremely socially harmful.

Plenty of depictions of humans absolutely feeling themselves exist from the ancient world. In spite of recent debates regarding the very existence of women's sexual pleasure, one of the oldest depictions of masturbation (dated to the fourth millennium BCE in Malta) is a clay figurine of a woman getting handsy with herself. Far more than just an activity to make you feel fierce and fine, masturbation served a social purpose in many cultures. The ancient Sumerians believed it would enhance one's sexual potency; the act could be carried out either alone or with one's chosen partner present—the OG act of mutual masturbation.

In ancient Egypt, wanking was thought responsible for perhaps the greatest social benefit imaginable—bringing the entire world into existence. Egyptian mythology told that the god Atum had created the universe by "nulling the void" in its most literal sense: the flow of the Nile River was even considered to be a result of the frequency of his ejaculations up in the heavens. To commemorate the most important secretion of bodily fluids of literally all time, Egyptian pharaohs wanked ceremonially into this river.

It is quite hard for us to imagine now, but there was a time when wrestling with your one-eyed wonder weasel was most likely considered only as scandalous as eating in public. The infamous philosopher Diogenes (died 320 BCE) provides a fantastic example. The founder of stoicism was renowned for his many public displays. These include but are far from limited to: bathing (as well as living) in a bathtub in the public agora, defecating in public, and wanking for all to see. In defense of his action, Diogenes is known to have stated, "If only it were as easy to banish hunger by rubbing one's belly." Interestingly, eating in the agora is listed among his social transgressions, suggesting that eating in public was likely considered as taboo as all the rest.

It seems our constantly changing relationship with bodily functions is far from limited to the philosophy of choking the chicken. We only have to look to the rules set by different cultures around the world to see the inconsistencies in how we relate to our bodies: to eat with your mouth open or closed, to use utensils or your hands, to hold in your burps or to slurp loudly during your meal. The differences we find across the globe should remind us that our thinking surrounding our bodies has *everything* to do with the influence of our social world. And particularly in the Western world, that influence can be summarized by one word: *shame*.

As we wine and dine, happily enjoying our gherkins and carrots, we are going to focus on the "kink" of pleasure. We will taste the decadent foods of twentieth-century America, Renaissance Italy, and the prehistoric era. We'll even try the long and storied flavors of the sex toys in your bedroom drawers: dildos, vibrators, and butt plugs. Strap yourself in—or on.

We will pause and savor the taste of eighteenth-century Europe the longest: this was our "war on masturbation," when we collectively decided it was a particularly shameful offense. Over the past few decades, we have made great progress in undoing those attitudes and transforming ourselves, slowly, into a more sex-positive society, but in many ways we are merely returning to an even older way of doing things.

Make yourself comfortable—this course is all about self-pleasure. Shame and stigma may be social phenomena, but masturbation and the use of sex toys are the ultimate statement of indulgence. They can correct the idea that we should be ashamed of ourselves and our bodies.

We are slowly turning into a society that learns how to prioritize pleasure for its own sake. But history doesn't always follow a set menu. Some prefer ordering off the à la carte menu, while others prefer eating their sweet before their savory . . .

Shall we dig in?

The War on Masturbation

One Hundred Hands of Solitude

I t is no coincidence that the words and phrases we use to describe masturbation are so odd and tonally undecided. As sex historian Dr. Kate Lister has observed:

> *As sex became repressed, words linking to the body became taboo. After all, how can we enjoy sexuality of our bodies, shame free, when the very words we use to talk about them, think about them or write about them are considered obscene?*

When it comes to self-pleasure, language can be incredibly medical and detached (autoeroticism, onanism, touching yourself), laden with violence and shame (self-abuse, self-pollution, beating the meat), or almost uncomfortably playful (hand party, playing with yourself, dueling with the pink Darth Vader). Even the term *masturbation* has a strange history. It was likely coined in 1712 by John Marten, an English surgeon who is believed to have written the widely influential publication *Onania; or, The Heinous Sin of Self-Pollution*. The tract sought to expose the "frightful consequences" faced by both sexes for engaging in any such act, which ranged from physical ailments to spiritual damnation.

This publication—and the plethora of similar publications it inspired—marks an important moment in the early modern period. It was during this time that our thinking relationship to a range of bodily functions (including sex, self-pleasure, and even eating) changed drastically. Masturbation had not needed a name prior to this moment because it was simply something that *happened*. The very act of naming masturbation was an attempt to police, not to understand, the behavior. Wanking was no longer something to enjoy in your bedchambers—now it was a diagnosis laden with shame.

Of course, no conversation about shameful masturbation would be complete without brief reference to everyone's favorite cerealist, Dr. John Harvey Kellogg (1852–1943). It is an endlessly fun fact for parties that Kellogg's Corn Flakes, a common product in pantries across the globe, were invented to stop people from masturbating. Kellogg was a proponent in the initial crusade against masturbation, claiming quite hilariously that "such a victim literally dies by his own hand." Engagements in such immoral acts of self-gratification would lead the sinful gratifier to develop . . . well, pretty much every ailment of which you could possibly think: vision loss, cancer of the womb, urinary diseases, nocturnal emissions, impotence, insanity, etc., etc.

In his publication *Plain Facts for Old and Young: Embracing the Natural History and Hygiene of Organic Life* (1887), Kellogg suggests a range of remedies for this plague on humanity: bandaging the hands of children or covering their genitals in cages before bedtime, and in the more extreme cases, sewing the foreskin shut or administering shock treatment. The publication reads more like a draft script for the *Saw* franchise than a manual for the medical treatment of young people.

In 1894, Kellogg was to release a widely accessible cure for this devilish epidemic—his cornflake cereal! Kellogg, like many others of this time, believed that flavorful food was responsible for increasing one's sexual libido; alternatively, bland food would help one stay grounded and away from passions. In comparison to today's product, Kellogg's original recipe was absent the one thing that makes the cereal bearable for consumption: sugar. But this wasn't his only food-based plan to curb sexual desire; around the same time, Kellogg experimented with a contraption that ran water through the bowel, following it with yogurt delivered to both the mouth and anus. This being the case, I think we should be somewhat grateful that the plain old cornflakes were the ones to catch on. Plus, they do taste wonderful when smothered in chocolate—a fantastic aphrodisiac, which we shall enjoy over dessert.

Let's remember that these views were happily published in magazines and on cereal boxes little more than one hundred years ago—and, as the continued existence of the Kellogg's brand attests, to some acclaim. Indeed, many of these anti-masturbatory attitudes have continued to hold sway over many of our lives. David Spiegelhalter has gone as far as to claim that the publication of *Onania* in 1712 "heralded a crushing attitude to masturbation that would last 250 years." In his fantastic overview of historical statistics regarding the practice, he points out that as late as the 1940s the United States Naval Academy, in Annapolis, had rules that stated candidates "shall be rejected by the examining surgeon for evidence of masturbation." Fears of resulting physical and spiritual ailments have remained alive and well this century; Katharine Davis's survey of women in 1929 proved a considerable portion still considered masturbation "morally degrading," and Masters and Johnson's study in the early 1960s showed many men still feared mental illness and "a case of nerves" as a result of excessively shaking hands with the milkman.

(Once we finish flicking our beans around the table, I will be sure to introduce you to these three eminent scientists!)

It is little wonder, then, that an ethos of shame still exists around acts of self-pleasure today. Even the most sex-positive members of our society have likely had to endure a process of unlearning cultural stigmas that persist around the act: it's shameful, it's dirty, it's something that should never be spoken of.

The result is far more than just a yucky feeling in your stomach after climaxing alone. How we talk and think about self-pleasure equally affects how we talk and think about sex—and we don't need to delve too deeply into our history books to see the danger of repressing that conversation. Just as acts of self-love were thought to play a beneficial role in times gone by, the same can be true today. Spiegelhalter states:

> *In response to current rates of teenage pregnancy and sexually transmitted diseases in young people, masturbation has come to be seen by some as a positive aspect of sexual health, encouraging awareness of sexuality in solitary safety and—now that blindness, insanity, clammy hands and pimples have finally been ruled out as side-effects—providing pleasure without associated risks.*

But how exactly did we move away from this default position of fear and shame surrounding sexuality that has plagued humanity for nearly 250 years?

Masters? Johnson? Are you ready? Ah, sticking right into the eggplant, I see. I think it's about time we discussed your research. James Joyce, you might want to prick your ears up for this one!

The (rather infamous) work of William H. Masters and Virginia E. Johnson was yet another important turning point in the history of sexuality; they performed their controversial trials in the second half of the twentieth century in the United States. They conducted a little bit more than just a paper survey—indeed, if we are going to discuss masturbation, then we really need to look to these researchers, who watched and recorded participants in the act of self-love, among many other things. Initially, their experiments were limited to paid sex workers, who, to the advantage of the research, were knowledgeable about sex and willing to cooperate with Masters and Johnson's peculiar requests. Later, the study expanded to 382 women and 312 men—albeit mostly white, educated, and married—allowing the researchers to conclude that they had observed "10,000 complete cycles of sexual response."

Now, the scenario was far from satin sheets and candlelight for the nearly one thousand participants, who were connected to instruments in the laboratory that would measure changes in their heart rate, breathing, and even their lubrication. And to preserve their anonymity, participants had the option to wear brown paper bags on their heads while the researchers recorded and observed their activities.

James Joyce is not the only one at this table inspired by a mythological battle with a cyclops from ancient Greece. For the purpose of the study, Masters and Johnson created "Ulysses," a whopping machine of a dildo with a camera placed inside to attain some "intravaginal photography." A bit different from your classic lewd picture, but I'll allow it. The primary achievement of this device was: (i) demonstration of how vaginal lubrication worked, dispelling previous beliefs that it originated from the cervix; and (ii) debunking the notion, popularized by Freud (we can't avoid him), that vaginal stimulation produced a superior orgasm to clitoral stimulation—an argument that had been used to demonstrate women's need for the Penis™. Ulysses proved once and for all that the orgasmic response was the same whether or not women decided to insert something inside.

Masters and Johnson became notorious because they became desensitized to their work. Admittedly, I have run into this same issue, forgetting after hours of reading about prehistoric dildos that not everyone considers this normal conversation in the faculty lounge. But I haven't gone quite as far as to display footage from an "intravaginal" photo shoot at a reputable academic seminar.

Yes, a video of a woman masturbating with Ulysses was played back to an audience of the duo's academic peers—a professional faux pas that saw them face increased scrutiny from said peers. Yet no slap on the wrist could smother their passion for the cause. When Masters and Johnson didn't have participants to complete their trials, they nobly took the burden upon themselves, engaging in erotic acts by themselves and with each other so they could continue their studies. For the sake of science.

Despite their questionable research practices (which *certainly* would not make it past ethics approval today), Masters and Johnson had a profound impact on sexual studies as we know them. The publication of their research, *Human Sexual Response*, in 1966 made a tremendous impact upon the legitimization of sexuality as a field for academic study, triggering a variety of further research. They rejected the idea of "sex exceptionalism"—that sex is an inherently different topic from other human activities. Indeed, by making it the focus of verifiable scientific observation, Masters and Johnson took sex and sexuality out of the Forbidden section of the academic library and demonstrated that this aspect of human life is part of our holistic well-being. Though Ulysses has (rightfully) gone to an early retirement, we remain indebted to their infamous contributions.*

---

* If you want to learn more, *Masters of Sex* (2013–16) is a period TV show dramatizing the work and relationship of Masters and Johnson, based on the 2009 biography of the same name by Thomas Maier.

The Birth of the Dildo

The history of the dildo far predates the birth of Ulysses—be that Ulysses the intravaginal photography machine, *Ulysses* the modernist literary masterpiece, or even the mythological Ulysses who fought the cyclops in ancient Greece.

Any reference to this topic needs to incorporate the work of Dr. Hallie Lieberman, who wrote one of the first PhD dissertations on the history of sex toys. Lieberman, welcome to our table!

The oldest known dildo has been dated to twenty-eight thousand years ago. For perspective, Lieberman points out we did not even invent writing until 3400–3100 BCE. Clearly, we were far more concerned about having orgasms than finding a means to document them. This incredible discovery was unearthed in 2005 as a team of researchers from Tübingen University explored the famous Hohle Fels cave, near Ulm in Germany's Swabian Jura region. It was here they discovered the final piece of their puzzle—the fourteen fragments of a twenty-centimeter-long, three-centimeter-wide siltstone object, destined to be the subject of much archaeological debate. However, the object's distinctive form, the etched rings around the tip, and the fact it was highly polished finally determined it was "a symbolic representation of male genitalia," the leading researcher, Professor Nicholas Conard, stated. Though it also bears scars typical of knapping flint, the primary use of this object was likely to start a wholly different kind of fire.

While this is the oldest known model to date, it is far from the only one of its kind: phallic batons have been found in Eurasia dated between 40,000 and 10,000 BCE; in a Mesolithic site in Motala, Sweden, from four thousand to six thousand years ago; and from a similar period in Pakistan; and sculptures of genitalia have been dated to the sixth century BCE in Turkey. Lieberman even discovered that double-ended dildos existed at least thirteen thousand to nineteen thousand years ago. "Sharing is caring" is an age-old sentiment.

One of the disadvantages of dildos being invented before writing, however, is that we don't have proof of how exactly they were used (I'm sure we can theorize that these penis miniatures sat on the sides of caves for "decorative" purposes). Yet we merely need to fast-forward a few centuries for confirmation.

In ancient Greece, dildos played a starring role. It was around this time that they really seemed to rise to popularity, as references to various instruments can be found in multiple mediums of art from that time. They were referred to as *olisbos*, from *olisthein*, which translated means "to slip or glide." The penis was highly symbolic in ancient Greece. As Paul Chrystal has poetically stated, "In the ancient world, generally, the penis was king, and masturbation was evidence of that regality." It held many different symbolic values: from strength and power to intellect and fertility. The Almighty Phallus, believe it or not, was an active participant in religious life, too—and had that stayed true, I may well have kept on at Sunday school. Aphrodite's temple was dressed to the nines with phalluses of all shapes and sizes. The largest dildos that ancient manufacturing would allow for were paraded through the cities by the cult of Dionysus—a practice not too dissimilar to a parade that still takes place in Japan.

Kanamara Matsuri, or the Festival of the Steel Phallus, is celebrated in April at Kanayama Shrine in Kawasaki. Its origins can be traced back to a rather interesting Shinto tale of a demon who decided to set up shop in a woman's vagina after falling madly in love with her (and you thought your ex had boundary issues). Utterly wracked with love and jealousy, this vagina-based demon decided to bite off the penis of the woman's suitor on their wedding night. After recovering from this traumatic attempted wedding, the woman would try to marry again—however, her second suitor would also be met with the same fate. (This is one of the many myths of *vagina dentata*—Latin for "toothed vagina"—that we can find across history.) And so, to secure herself a far more successful wedding night the *third* time, the woman commissioned a blacksmith to create an iron phallus. Taking matters literally into her own hand, she used this iron dildo to defeat the demon—breaking its teeth and ultimately destroying it after it tried to take a chomp. This lifesaving dildo was thus enshrined in Kanayama.

The shrine is now the location of Kawasaki's annual Penis Festival, in the greater Tokyo area—and the day really lives up to its name. The festival is filled with penis-shaped everything: penis-shaped lollipops, penis-shaped costumes, penis-shaped hats—and, of course, the giant penises that are proudly paraded down the city streets. In essence, the day celebrates fertility and the creation of life—in other words, sex. Between the seventeenth and nineteenth centuries, the Kanayama shrine was a popular place for sex workers to leave offerings and prayers to protect themselves from sexually transmitted diseases, just as the tale's heroine was protected after taking back control of her body. It was around this time that the small-scale festival, which focuses on sexual health, became linked to this location. Yet, it was not until the 1970s that it was revived as a tradition, and within only a few years, it had truly taken off. The event today is connected to a celebration of sex-positive and LGBTQIA+ advocacy—a day of public pride and expression of identity and sexuality. And it all started with one woman's lifesaving iron dildo.

This is far from the only ancient tale in which a woman uses a dildo to achieve liberation. To return to ancient Greece, the dildo plays a leading role in Aristophanes's comedy *Lysistrata* (411 BCE). This Greek play tells the story of how a group of creative women endeavor to end the Peloponnesian War by denying their men the one thing they truly desire: a special cuddle for grown-ups. Lysistrata encourages the women of the warring cities to go on a sex strike, denying their husbands and lovers any sexual favors until they agree to start negotiating peace. And to quell their own desire, Lysistrata encourages the women to use their "eight-fingered leather dildos . . . as a sort of flesh-replacement for our poor cunts." The women seal this oath around a bowl of wine, swearing to opt for their dildos over men (which honestly just sounds like a fantastic Saturday night).

A multifaceted actor, the dildo also appears in the sixth mime of Herodas (third century BCE). This performance features a heated discussion between a group of women about who gets to borrow a coveted dildo next. This specific bedroom aid has proven itself superior to those sold by other makers: "Hunt as you might, you will not find another cobbler so kindly disposed to women." In fact, this dildo proves itself to be not only the favorite of the toys,* but even superior to the thing itself: "The men certainly have no rams like those."

At this time, it is also rumored that dildos began to . . . go against the grain. In fact, around the year 5 BCE, a special breadstick was reportedly made for bedroom pleasure. This has been called an *olisbokollix* (ὀλισβοκόλλιξ)—the ancient Greek term *kollix* refers to bread; *olisbos*, as mentioned, refers to dildo. Surviving vases depict the object in question, and the word appears in the richly complicated lexicon of Hesychius of Alexandria—indicating that if not real, there was at the very least a widely spread joke about its existence, thus confirming a general knowledge of sexual aids.

This isn't the only instance of the ancient Greeks cooking up a storm in the bedroom. Olive oil was a popular form of lubrication,† and whatever brand they were using, it definitely wasn't extra virgin. The earliest written record of its use dates back to 350 BCE. Aristotle advised in *The History of Animals*, book VII, part 3, that pregnancy could be prevented by ensuring the woman's "womb" did not come into contact with the man's sperm; this could be achieved by rubbing it with cedar oil, lead ointment, or incense, mixed with olive oil.‡ As well as solving the issue of unwanted pregnancy and aiding men to slip into tight places, olive oil was generously smeared on dildos, which were commonly made from wood or pressed leather, before use. Olive oil became a treasure throughout the ancient world—the pots that contained it were beautifully decorated, most often with highly erotic art. Surviving pots depict everything from homosexuality and cross-dressing to group activities and depictions of these breadstick dildos being put to good use.

Despite this apparent openness, there were still strict rules for how dildos could be used—closely related to the rules concerning same-sex activity. As penetration was

---

* I think there's great potential for a *Toy Story* sequel set in Andy's mom's room.

† As women's health expert Dr. Sherry A. Ross noted in *Men's Health* in 2019, olive oil is still a surprisingly popular option for lubrication today: "Long ago, olive oil was readily available, effective and a natural lubricant. In the modern age, olive oil is still used as a viable and popular sexual lubricant." See Kim Wong-Shing, "A Brief History of Lube, from 350 BCE Onward," *Men's Health*, April 3, 2019, https://menshealth.com/sex-women/a27017053/history-of-lube-sex/.

‡ DO NOT try this one at home.

deemed a masculine act, it was considered shameful for men to allow themselves to be penetrated with any sesame-seeded baguettes. Women were, it seems, free to use dildos among themselves. Remaining artwork from the time depicts dildos in use during both homosexual acts between women as well as masturbation (mutual or solo).

It would well be worth pausing here to mention one of my favorite facts of all time. *Lysistrata* may not be the oldest literary reference on record of the dildo—that may actually come from the Bible. When I read this fact in Lieberman's *Buzz: The Stimulating History of the Sex Toy* (2017), I damn near threw the book across the room. Of all the books in the world, the Holy Bible was the last place I expected to find sex toys. Somehow, after spending so long studying the saucy secrets of the past, even I can be surprised. In the Old Testament, Ezekiel 16:17, God reprimands the people of Jerusalem because they "took the gold and silver" that he had given them and made "phallic images and fornicated with them." These objects are believed to have referred to dildos (because honestly, what else could "phallic images" made for fornicating *be*?). Around the time I found out about this fact and blasted it on the internet, I was informed that unicorns also make an appearance in the Bible. If only the fun parts of the Good Book had featured in Religious Studies.

Soon after my video was posted, I received a notification that Dr. Dan McClellan, theologian and scripture translator, had made a video in response. My heart was beating out of my chest. This was it, I thought. This was the day my credibility was derided on the internet. With my pulse beating so fast that my smartwatch thought I was doing intense exercise, I pressed play . . .

And I lived to see another day on the internet! There was, in fact, truth to this interpretation. McClellan explained that the original verb used to describe this fornication is *zanah*, which is often used in a metaphorical sense in the Hebrew Bible to refer to worshipping other deities—symbolically committing adultery against the God of Israel. While this passage could thus be read as a metaphorical fornication with "phallic images," McClellan said it is also plausible to interpret this passage literally. The book of Ezekiel features a number of sexually shocking moments, so it's likely the people of Israel were depicted to be fornicating with dildos as a way of illustrating how depraved they had become.

Dildos in ancient Egypt played a different role. Typically made of stone and leather, they were a multitalented companion, celebrated for their ability to provide sexual pleasure, and thus found a use in ritual, religious, and even magical practices. Erotic art from the time depicts men and women alike reaping the benefits. Due to their close association with spirituality, dildos were also used as funerary objects, and have been discovered in excavated tombs. Even the deceased deserved access to their favorite bedroom toys.

A similar story is found in the history of ancient China's Han Dynasty. As Jay Xu, director of the Asian Art Museum of San Francisco, stated in a widely cited interview:

> *The Han, like the Egyptians, also conceived of a soul dualism, or a vital essence, one on earth in the body (po) and one in the ethereal beyond (hun), that could linger on into eternity—even immortality . . . as long as it was properly cared for, and you had the right funerary rites, and regalia and retinue to keep the spirit alive and entertained, and also adequately nourished after death.*

As spirits were believed to live inside tombs, it was therefore important for them to be buried with the objects that had been precious during their life—such as their dildos. Sexuality played an important role in the Han Dynasty. The passionate act of sex was believed to bring the forces of yin and yang into balance, a powerful experience that could momentarily raise a person's consciousness to the plane of life and death. This made access to sex toys crucial if the deceased did awaken to find themselves trapped within the tomb—the dildo would basically act as their one-way ticket to the higher plane. Museum curators of these items are all in agreement that they were not merely for decorative purposes:

> *They were all definitely made for use, and we can speculate based on their various bases how they were worn. They're all bespoke, and the ones we have here might have been laced into place with leather or silk thongs, though it's not clear if they were designed for men or women—they're not heavy at all— though the phallus without the ring form was likely for a man since it was found in a king's tomb.*

Dildos weren't the only spicy toys found in these tombs—archaeologists have also found butt plugs in their midst. These, however, were likely used for a little more work and a lot less play, used to seal the body and maintain its qi, the vital essence that can leak out of the body during life and death. This isn't dissimilar to A/V plugs used by morticians today to keep fluids from leaking out of a deceased body. Most people don't know that you could well be buried with an anal/vaginal plug, but it's true. So, why wait until you're dead?

While jade butt plugs might have fallen out of fashion, the dildo remained popular throughout the early modern period; we continue to find references to everyone's favorite bedfellow in art and literature. The forefather of pornography, Pietro Aretino (1492–1556), often wrote about dildos, particularly in the more . . . unexpected places. In *Ragionamenti* (1534), there is a particularly amusing episode in which the character of Nana describes a basket of glass dildos being delivered in the middle of a gathering.

> *Then he uncovered his basket and set it on the table. At once a roar of laughter arose that sounded like thunder. No sooner were those fruits of paradise seen than the hands of both sexes, already engaged with one another's thighs, tits, flutes and bags, lunged for them with the dexterity of pickpockets. . . . They were glass fruits made in Murano near Venice to look like a prick.*

It is fair to say that the "glass fruits" referenced here looked far closer to a glass vegetable, namely, an eggplant. Indeed, Aretino would refer to these coveted toys in his work as *pastinaca muranese*, which has been translated to "crystal turnip." By 1598, the use of this phrase had become so common, due to Aretino, that it was granted its own entry in Florio's Italian–English dictionary—translated officially there as "a dildoe made of glasse."

At this time, Venice was the center of luxurious dildo production. The dildos were fashioned from fine Venetian glass and designed to be filled with warm water to simulate the feeling of real ejaculation. Aretino also wrote about the use of dildos by nuns. In *Ragionamenti* (which has been translated to *The Secret Lives of Nuns*) we read about a nun putting one of these self-ejaculating dildos to use to "quell the gnawing of the flesh." One of these ejaculating dildos, dated to the eighteenth century, was discovered at the old site of a convent, hidden in the seat of a Louis XV armchair, near the banks of the Seine in France. This discovery confirms that these lifelike dildos were far more than just a figment of the literary imagination.

Having now ticked off Italy and France, we can also find evidence of dildos in England. Even Shakespeare had something to say. When you were studying the great bard in English class, I would wager your teacher may have forgotten to mention the traveling dildo salesman—but there he is. In act III of *The Winter's Tale*, a servant describes a peddler he has seen selling some truly interesting wares:

> *He hath songs for man or woman, of all sizes; no milliner can so fit his customers with gloves. He has the prettiest love songs for maids, so without bawdry, which is strange with such delicate burdens of dildos and fadings, "Jump her and thump her"; and where some stretch-mouthed rascal would, as it were, mean mischief and break a foul gap into the matter, he makes the maid to answer, "Whoop, do me no harm, good man"; puts him off, slights him, with "Whoop, do me no harm, good man!"*

"Fadings" in this context isn't quite as innocent as it may sound. It was another term for "dying," which was a common Elizabethan way of speaking about orgasming. I originally believed this came from the French phrase *la petite mort* ("the little death"), which is also a euphemism for orgasm, but according to the *Oxford English Dictionary*, this did not come into use in this context until the nineteenth century.

The origin of both euphemisms for climax may actually come from the dominant logic behind Renaissance medicine. The theory of humorism originated in the works of Hippocrates and was widely accepted in ancient Greece and Rome, as well as in medieval Europe. It guided the practice of medicine for over two thousand years and didn't fall out of favor until well into the nineteenth century.

Basically, we believed that the body was made of four humors, or bodily fluids: blood (*haima*), phlegm (*phlegma*), yellow bile (*xanthe chole*), and black bile (*melaina chole*). Yum! Disease and illness were caused by imbalance of these humors. This theory was entwined with the study of astrology. The time of year you were born decided the humor that most dominated your body, and physicians would use astrological charts to make diagnoses and to select treatments. It is also why bloodletting was a common treatment for illness and disease. You may have seen this in historical fiction TV shows—leeches are placed, or a vein is briefly opened, to relieve the "humors" that have built up in this area.

When people reached climax, it was thought that they drained out their bodily fluids (i.e., humors). Depending on which source you go to, this was a good or bad thing. Orgasm became known as "dying" because it released vital life fluids, and too much of a good thing could well bring you to the point of death. However, some historians have suggested this logic was actually used to *encourage* people to have sex; similar to the practice of bloodletting, humors could thus be released from the body to prevent them from building up. In particular, if you found yourself infatuated, humors would build up in your genitals, and sex was a healthy way to regulate their dispersion.

The humorous (see what I did there?) interlude in *The Winter's Tale*, which is easy to miss, is one of the first uses of the word *dildo* in the English language. Another writer, however, got in first. Written around 1592, "The Choise of Valentines or the Merie Ballad of Nash His Dildo" is an erotic poem by Thomas Nash (and also referred to as "Nash's Dildo"). In this piece, we are introduced to a dildo of "thick congealed glasse" that is able to be filled "with whott water, or with milk" to squirt into the user.

In the poem, we can also observe a shifting cultural perspective that begins to link the dildo to anxieties of emasculation. On Valentine's Day, our hero, Tomalin, travels out to the country to enjoy some typically Valentiney activity with his lover, Mistress Frances. However, he discovers upon arrival that she now lives in a brothel in the city. By the time he has made his way there (and negotiated with the brothel madame, who offers him every other worker before allowing him access to Mistress Frances), Tomalin is so excited by the journey that he ejaculates almost as soon as he sees his love before him.

Oh, who is able to abstaine so long?
I com! I com!

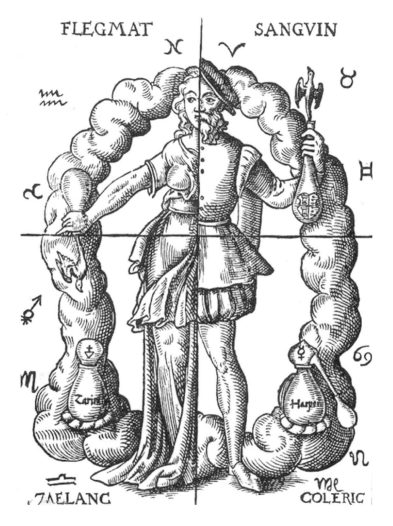

FLEGMAT   SANGVIN

ZAELANG   COLERIC

An illustration in Leonhard Thurneisser zum Thurn's scholarly text *Quinta Essentia* (1574) depicts the concept of the four humors in relation to the four elements and signs of the zodiac.

Unhappy that her lover has finished before her fun has even begun, Mistress Frances lends a "helping hand" to help get her lover back in the mood.

"Unhappie me," quoth shee, "and wil't not stand?
Com, lett me rubb and chafe it with my hand!"

Tomalin is once again ready for action . . . only to prematurely ejaculate once more. Mistress Frances gives up all hopes of a satisfactory interaction and takes hold of her "little dilldo." The rest of the poem consists of her singing the praises of the dildo over a man, for it always "stands as stiff as he were made of steele," and does not run the risk of pregnancy—making her "tender bellie swell." All the while Tomalin watches on, humiliated and defeated by his artificial opponent.

What Nash's poem indicates (along with the dangers of a prolonged train ride) is the shifting connection of sex toys to cultural fears of emasculation. Indeed, by the end of the seventeenth century, feelings toward these alternative bedfellows were really starting to change across Europe. We need only ask the notorious Earl of Rochester, John Wilmot, to tell us all about it. He is that rakish libertine at the other end of the table, hogging the wine and commanding everyone's attention as he recites his poetry.

Cupid and Bacchus my saints are,
May drink and love still reign,
With wine I wash away my cares,
And then to cunt again!

Wilmot was known for his bawdy and satirical poetry, as well as the sexually promiscuous lifestyle he led during the Restoration period in England. His debaucheries included hosting wild parties and orgies at his estate, engaging in innumerable extramarital affairs with both men and women, and "donating" his services to infertile couples who were struggling to conceive. A very generous man. He also dabbled as a gynecologist, playing dress-up and adopting the persona of "Dr. Bendo"; some of his patients even decided to keep him on after his fraudulence was revealed.

In 1670, Wilmot placed a large order of dildos for one of his sex parties, but they never made it and were instead seized by English customs and all the party favors burned. Understandably, Wilmot wasn't too happy about his Amazon Prime order going up in flames and, as the seventeenth-century version of leaving a bad Google review, published a poem in response: "Signior Dildo."

You Ladyes all of Merry England
Who have been to kisse the Dutchesse's hand,
Pray did you lately observe in the Show
A Noble Italian call'd Signior Dildo? . . .
You'll take him at first for no Person of Note
Because he appears in a plain Leather Coat:
But when you his virtuous Abilities know
You'll fall down and Worship Signior Dildo.

That is quite enough, Wilmot, but thank you for leading us in that roaring song.

The poem, quite amusingly, personifies the dildo into a strapping Italian lover. The immense "discretion and vigor" of Signior Dildo is far superior to the lovers the ladies of England have otherwise known. If we think back to Nash's ballad, we can really see male anxiety coming into play. Men may be good, but women will "fall down and Worship Signior Dildo." Unless, of course, you're Dr. Bendo, and excessively confident in your capabilities as a lover.

But why an Italian lover? Well, as Lieberman has pointed out, Italy was the largest purveyor of dildos in Europe. Other writers, such as Jack Holland, have theorized this cultural divide could well be responsible for the shift of opinion: "For an Englishman, what could be more humiliating than to be superannuated by an Italian dildo?" The fear of emasculation is therefore linked to cultural tensions in Europe. As a result, importation of sex toys into England and France became increasingly difficult—so much so that women across Europe began to find their own solutions, making and selling bedroom companions themselves. #BossBitchBehavior. It became so widespread that in England laws were written to ban women from creating dildos for themselves or each other.

Teresia Constantia Phillips (1709–1765), whom we had the honor of meeting earlier this evening, owned the Green Canister on Half Moon Street in the Strand, stocked to the brim with everything to satisfy your needs. Mrs. Phillips's shop was renowned. References to it can be found in a variety of items from the period. For instance, the satirical print *A Sale of English Beauties in the East-Indies* (1786), now displayed in the

British Museum, depicts a range of items going up for auction—including a box of rods of "British Manufacture" designed for sexual flagellation, as well as one labeled from Mrs. Phillips in Leicester Square.

As well as encouraging safer practices of sex, as we heard earlier, Mrs. Phillips curated a notable variety of dildos. For a price between two and ten pounds, one could purchase whichever one best suited one's desire—be it one made from Indian rubber or a double-ended item, "one that can be used by two."

Unfortunately, the dildo finds itself implicated by the War on Masturbation, which really heats up around the beginning of the eighteenth century. Though fun ditties and odes to the dildo appear in publication, the use of sex toys becomes increasingly vilified, with the threat of prosecution. For that reason, the next major event in the life of the dildo would not take place for a couple of centuries. Flash forward to the 1960s, where we are met with the incredible, if often forgotten, contributions of Gosnell Duncan, whose story has been brought to light by Hallie Lieberman. While working at the International Harvester Company in Chicago in 1965, Duncan, a Grenadian immigrant, was injured and paralyzed from the waist down. The accident left him impotent, and it became apparent to him that he could not easily find a safe penile substitute.

> *As I was learning to live my life from scratch, no one even mentioned the word "sexuality."*

Despite the fact they *were* sold as medical aids, dildos at the time were low quality and made of rubber. This meant they couldn't withstand heat or washing—two pretty important factors when it comes to sanitization. Duncan decided to take matters into his own hands. He worked with a chemist to create the silicone dildo, hoping to provide a better and safer option for people with a disability. It took off, and the silicone dildo soon became the immensely popular and inclusive toy we know today.*

---

* I encourage you to read the rest of Duncan's story in more detail (Lieberman's writing and research into his biography are truly admirable).

Definitions of Pleasure

T wenty-eight thousand years after their first known appearance, it is fair to say that dildos and sex toys are still very much in use. Our survey recorded that 73.7 percent of participants had used a sex toy. These numbers can't simply be explained by the younger generation (who were the dominant demographic on this survey) being more open. In fact, the highest frequency of sex-toy use came from the thirty to thirty-nine age bracket, followed by participants aged forty to forty-nine years. By far, the highest category of people making use of bedroom toys was those with a postgraduate university degree—80.6 percent. On the other end of the spectrum, those with less than a high school degree were the lowest-scoring, with less than half (49.04 percent) claiming they had ever used a toy during an act of self-love.

Education has been shown to affect masturbation rates in general. It seems the higher your level of education, the more likely you are to enjoy a little procrastination in the bedroom (writing doctoral theses is a long and boring process, OK?).* This is also far from a new finding—let's talk about the groundbreaking research into women's sexuality by Katharine Bement Davis (1860–1935), an American social reformer and criminologist.

There she is, near the head of the table! It seems Davis is engrossed in conversation with Virginia Woolf at present, discussing everything from women's suffrage to child

* In the previous year, 47.1 percent of women with a post–high school education masturbated, compared with 29.5 percent of women who didn't graduate high school; the figures for men were 73 percent compared with 64.5 percent. This data is from the latest national Australian Study of Health and Relationships, in 2014.

welfare. Even in the midst of a lively and stimulating conversation, however, Davis never loses sight of her impeccable manners and grace, and her presence here is a true delight to all who have the pleasure of sitting with her.

While she is so deeply engrossed in her conversation, I really must tell you all about her work. In 1929, Davis published data she had collected from questionnaires sent out to twenty thousand women from local organizations and college alumni registers. The findings were scandalous, demonstrating that (*shock! horror!*) women do actually have a libido. While we are right to consider them biased now, the results from this group of white educated women are interesting to compare with the reported results from other women of the time.

Davis's study showed that 60 percent of unmarried women reported they'd enjoyed "womansplaining themselves" and 30 percent of married respondents had done so prior to marriage (presumably they were expected to stop now that they had access to the Almighty Penis). Even compared with the 42 percent reported today, that number is *wild*, let alone in comparison with what other studies were finding at the time. Contrast this number with results of a study conducted by Simon Szreter and Kate Fisher of people born between 1901 and 1931:* out of fifty-seven women, only two people reported that they had ever self-pleasured, while seven claimed they did not know that such an act even existed. Education—and, in particular, *access* to education—plays a crucial role in influencing the relationship we have to our sexuality. Recent national surveys have *also* found a direct correlation between higher education and higher rates of masturbatory activities, especially those that incorporate sex toys. When we take into consideration the significant obstacles placed—even today—in the way of women accessing education, it is really no wonder that reported rates of masturbation remain so low.

There is one particularly interesting finding from the second British *National Survey of Sexual Attitudes and Lifestyles* (2003). The researchers reported that increased sexual activity in women was associated with increased masturbation—while for men, the opposite was true. The authors stated:

---

* I am indebted to Spiegelhalter for placing these two studies in direct comparison within his own work to draw attention to the inconstancy of the reported figures.

It is difficult to avoid the conclusion that masturbation for many predominately heterosexual men may represent a substitute for vaginal sex, while for women the practice appears to be part of the wider repertoire of sexual fulfillment, supplementing, rather than compensating for, partnered sex among women.

I can almost see it now—Sigmund Freud, in his grave, tearing out his hair (it does continue to grow after you die) and cursing for the umpteenth time the eternal mystery that is women's sexuality. *Women!* Will you never be satisfied? A whole minute and a half with a bloke in the bed and yet you *still* feel the need for a buzz in the bathroom.

Freudian breakdown aside, this conclusion is genuinely fascinating. That sex plays such an influential role not only in our capacity for pleasure but also in the very structure of pleasure itself is such an underestimated and yet interesting conversation in itself. How can we begin to talk about and report acts of self-pleasure when we don't even understand what pleasure is?

The Pleasure Principle

I t seems to me that pleasure is structured in distinctive ways. Pleasure can be linear, a gradual rise toward euphoric release that finally settles into a state of rest. In other cases, it is circular: a regenerative force constantly invigorated by the energy poured into it. Maybe it could be that women's experience of pleasure is more often structured as the latter—and instead of trying to understand this throughout history, we have just been maddened by its inability to fit neatly into a linear structure.

I am not the first person to make this observation. In 1997, Beverly Whipple and Karen Brash-McGreer proposed a circular model of women's sexual responses. The four stages—seduction (desire), sensations (excitement and plateau), surrender (orgasm), and reflection (resolution)—don't all need to happen, nor do they need to happen in that order. This means that a woman can feel desire, become aroused, and feel satisfaction without having an orgasm.

Three years later, Rosemary Basson would suggest another circular model: emotional intimacy, sexual stimuli, sexual arousal, arousal and sexual desire, and emotional and physical satisfaction. These all form a circle around the "spontaneous sexual drive." What was novel about Basson's research was that it indicated that women generally need to be aroused prior to becoming interested in sex—and there are many ways for this to happen. It can be caused by physical touch, seeing people kiss, or stumbling across Barbie pornography on YouTube (patience, dear reader—all will be revealed). The other factor she believed often, though not always, distinguishes women's sexual experience is the *motivation* for the sexual behavior. Men generally see sex as an end in itself, whereas for women, it's more commonly seen as a means to something else—whether that's greater emotional intimacy with a partner, a stress relief, or the pleasurable feelings it brings about.

Perhaps because of this complexity, women are generally more creative when it comes to beating around the bush. Indeed, women who have masturbated in the past year are five times more likely to have done so with a sex toy or other sexual aid than men.* If we are to take the confusion over the definition of masturbation into consideration, we may likely already see a closing of the gap when it comes to self-pleasure. This may help us to understand the regularly quoted statistic that men masturbate twice as often as women. This fact has been proven fairly consistently across national surveys conducted in Australia, the UK, and the USA.† In Britain's third *National Survey of Sexual Attitudes and Lifestyles* (2013), 66 percent of men and 33 percent of women reported to have self-pleasured in the previous four weeks. Comparably, the Australian Study of Health and Relationships in 2014 found 72 percent of men enjoyed this pastime in the previous twelve months compared with 42 percent of women. The fact that men are more frequently going at it alone may not be overly shocking.

However, it is not quite as easy to boil down these statistics to the assumption that one half of the population is naturally more horned up than the other. There are several reasons why the (reported) figures of women enjoying a little *ménage à moi* appear comparatively lower.

One not-so-apparent reason is that there is no definitive definition of "female masturbation." Some researchers have pointed toward the complexity of the woman's orgasm perhaps accounting for this gap in self-gratification. Just like with *sex*, there seems to be a range of definitions floating around when it comes to fEmAlE mAsTuRbAtIoN.

---

* Twenty-four percent of women in 2014 used sex toys, compared with 16 percent of men. Sourced from Richard O. de Visser et al., "Change and Stasis in Sexual Health and Relationships: Comparisons between the First and Second Australian Studies of Health and Relationships," *Sexual Health* 11, no. 5 (2014): 505–9, https://doi.org/10.1071/SH14112.

† I will importantly flag here, before discussion of these surveys continues, that one of the failings of these studies (more obvious to us now) is the strict adherence to the use of gender binaries. The experiences of those who did not fit within a tidy pink or blue pigeonhole have unfortunately been left out—meaning that the results can hardly be considered an encompassing snapshot. Moreover, it also flags how prevalent beliefs about gender influence even "objective" studies.

Australian researchers became aware of this discrepancy when gathering data for the national survey. There was no collective understanding of what masturbation actually was: Did it only include internal penetration? Did external stimulation count? Did you need to experience an orgasm? And what about setting your washing machine on spin mode if you just happened to be sitting there? How we account for "female masturbation" in studies is just not as straightforward as the male equivalent; for instance, it's uncommon for a man to enjoy a little alone time with his dominant hand and not "finish," whereas this scenario seems more common (and not necessarily disagreeable) to many women.

The simplicity with which we classify these gender-binary definitions of masturbation demands reexamination. If our experience of pleasure were in any way simple, then many hours—indeed years—of research would have been avoided (and it likely would not have become one of the most—if not the most—popular experiences for industries to capitalize upon). Treating the pleasure experience of any human as an unexacting journey from A to B will get us no further than those letters in the alphabet. The pleasure of all people has nuance, has complexities, has stories.

The fact that difficulty defining masturbation isn't just an exclusive issue of one demographic has come to the attention of wider research. One paper from 2018 demonstrated confusion across the board. In this study, 48.9 percent of men and 38.2 percent of women reported they would say they had masturbated if they had touched or stimulated their *partner's* genitals—an act that involved no direct pleasure for them. This finding is significant—nearly half of the male participants believed that the act of masturbation was different from its accepted definition as solo play. The researchers concluded that future studies needed to ask very specific questions, as "the term masturbation does not have one universal definition but rather encompasses many different behaviors for different individuals."

It was for this reason that we provided a precise list of definitions on our survey—to provide clarification as well as a more nuanced definition of pleasure than *Did you rub one out?* The numbers we drew up were a whole lot different from the previous 72:42 male-to-female ratio. In fact, a whopping 96.4 percent of our participants said they had masturbated by themselves in the past year. Males had the highest rate of participation at 99.1 percent, followed by nonbinary people at 96.3 percent. While the vast majority claimed to have masturbated in the past year, there was a notable difference in frequency. Nearly a quarter of males (22.7 percent) said they had masturbated more than once daily over the previous four weeks, compared with 5 percent of females, whereas nearly a quarter of women (24.2 percent) said they had masturbated less than once per week, compared with 7.5 percent of males.

As we know all too well, the subject of women's autonomous pleasure has repeatedly been met with debate, denial, or indifference. If you shake the majority of history books, a gaggle of sexless women is likely to fall out upon your lap (fixing their petticoats, fainting, and declaring *Oh, my!*). A trope that always amuses me in historical romance fiction—if we are allowed to get to the juicy bit—is the sexual awakening of the virtuous heroine on her wedding night to the story's hero (who has likely stopped brooding at this point and has proven himself to be a good guy, really). We do take it entirely for granted that the hands of our historical women never, perchance, felt the need to stray, that they were never moved to scratch an itch and then thought to themselves, *Why stop there?* The Sexless Woman is still spotted far too frequently in our envisionings of history, before she somehow woke up in the 1970s and realized she had a clitoris. There is no story, I believe, that captures this vision more quintessentially than the ill-told tale of how the vibrator was invented.

The Vibrator

Good Vibes Only

I t is possible that you have previously come across the shocking story of how the vibrator was invented. The story goes that in nineteenth-century Britain, "hysterical" women suffering chronic anxiety were prescribed pelvic finger massage. However, this was taking such a toll on the doctors' poor hands that they invented something to do the job for them. This story has made its way into TV shows (such as a recent episode of the animated sitcom *Big Mouth*) and plays, and has even been the focus of Hollywood movies such as the 2011 film *Hysteria*, starring Maggie Gyllenhaal. In fact, it has become so ingrained in pop culture that even when sex historian Hallie Lieberman published compelling evidence that completely debunked this version of history, she barely made a dent. This is a shame, not only because it's inaccurate but also because the true story is far more interesting—and far more feminist.

To weed out the fact from the fiction, we as always need to start back in the ancient world. Let me introduce you to the theory of the wandering womb. This was the belief that a woman's uterus occasionally became restless and just liked to go for a little stroll around the body. The earliest written record of this less than scientific theory can be found in the gynecological treatise of the *Hippocratic Corpus*, "Diseases of Women" (fifth to fourth century BCE). A wandering womb could result in a variety of ailments—mental, physical, and emotional. The symptoms were dependent on which area of the body the uterus had decided to wander off to. This condition was named after one of the Greek words for the uterus, *hystera*. Another physician, Aretaeus, described it thus:

> *In the middle of the flanks of women lies the womb, a female viscus, closely*
> *resembling an animal; for it is moved of itself hither and thither in the flanks,*
> *also upward in a direct line to below the cartilage of the thorax, and also*
> *obliquely to the right or to the left, either to the liver or the spleen, and it like-*
> *wise is subject to prolapsus downwards, and in a word, it is altogether erratic.*
> *It delights also in fragrant smells, and advances toward them; and it has an*
> *aversion to fetid smells, and flees from them; and, on the whole, the womb is*
> *like an animal within an animal.*

Why was it that, of all the parts of the human body, this specific organ had difficulty staying still? Was it rebellion? Boredom? Plain old womanly deviance? We encounter some difference in opinion. Hippocrates's texts theorized that the issue was thirst—the womb would wander around the body in search of more fluid. Alternatively, Soranus of Ephesus (the second-century physician) proposed an alternative idea, "hysterical suffocation," which had lasting implications: "The uterus does not issue forth like a wild animal from the lair, delighted by fragrant odors and fleeing bad odors, rather it is drawn together because of stricture caused by inflammation."

The concept of a condition called *hysteria* caused by the wandering womb—which is often heard about through its supposed connection to the invention of the vibrator—developed from this idea, most importantly in Edward Jorden's work *A Briefe Discourse of a Disease Called the Suffocation of the Mother* (1603). It was here that the wandering womb was popularized as a concept in early modern Europe and hysteria used as an explanation for mysterious medical occurrences in young women. In fact, Jorden went so far as to suggest that these pesky restless wombs could be the source of witchcraft.

By the end of the seventeenth century, however, the popularized condition of hysteria ceased to be linked to the world of witchcraft and wizardry. Instead, it became a medical issue—one treated surprisingly similarly to its management in ancient Greece. The behavioral deviance that characterized hysteria was once again thought to be caused by retention of fluids in the uterus, sexual deprivation, and, stop me if you've heard this, the tendency of the uterus to go gallivanting around the body. As a medical issue, it was given medically prescribed cures.

Let's get one thing straight—masturbation was *not* one of the prescribed cures for female hysteria. That simply would have been too much fun. This was a patriarchal disease and thus needed a patriarchal cure—sex with one's husband. *This* was the cure recommended to women who were acting "hysterical." In fact, marriage and regular sexual encounters with one's husband were considered the only long-term solution, and masturbation was believed to *worsen* the effects. Although hysteria was thought to be the result of built-up fluid within the uterus that needed to be regularly expelled, the uterus then benefited from being filled with the "healing properties" supposedly found only in a man's semen.

Honestly, this kind of "science" sounds like something you'd hear on "alpha male" podcasts today.

For this reason, not only was self-pleasure considered dangerous to women, contraceptive practices were, too. The one true cure for women's irrationality and irritability was not masturbation or condoms—it was marriage and childbearing. And if pleasure was derived from this (which, without a doubt, it would be, being women's destined purpose on this earth), then a woman's hysteria would be cured for good. If these women remained unmarried—by choice or circumstance—certain ministrations from midwives could aid the treatment of hysteria, such as stimulation of the area with oils and scents to release the fluid. However, this was, importantly, considered to be a last resort—and, in itself, not so much a cure as a Band-Aid on the issue. Only the power of semen could truly save women from themselves.

Now, I claim no medical qualifications, but if I am given leave to offer my opinion on the matter, it is that this sounds like a "disease" that had less to do with women's health and more to do with (men's) control over women and their bodies.

So how and why did vibrators become associated with this rather bleak story? We are brought to a tipping point in the nineteenth century when we made a hobby out of labeling things—like homosexuality, bisexuality, and other forms of "sexual deviance"—and turning these labels into diagnoses. (We will look much more closely at this tipping point over our next course.) Men began to consider hysteria more of a psychological ailment than a physical one. The stress of the modern, industrialized world was too much for a delicate woman's nerves, causing a variety of psychological disorders, not to mention increasingly faulty reproductive tracts. To calm the body and nerves, massage treatments from physicians were believed to have been practiced—and this is where our misconceptions emerge. In 1999, technology historian Rachel Maines *hypothesized* that hysteria may have been treated via the stimulation of the female's genitals, and that the time consumption and general inconvenience of this therapy led to technological advancements in the field. Cue the vibrator.

Despite its stubborn persistence in pop culture and the media, this claim has been widely disputed by multiple historians, most prominently in the work of Hallie Lieberman. While Lieberman agrees there is evidence that Victorian doctors used vibrators to treat hundreds of diseases at the time—including hysteria—no claims were made that vibrators could *cure* these aliments. What's more, she debunks the idea that vibrators were ever intended for clitoral stimulation. *Au contraire*, physicians were deterred from placing them anywhere near this sensitive area. In fact, the original vibrator wasn't even necessarily intended for women, let alone hysterical ones.

In the early 1880s, the first electric vibrator was invented by a physician, the British doctor Joseph Mortimer Granville. And this device was for men.

The vibrator was invented to cure a variety of ailments, such as spinal disease, deafness, and general bodily pain. As Lieberman has demonstrated, the only thing close to a suggestion of sexual use comes from its role in curing impotence, wherein the device was positioned to vibrate against the man's perineum. The vibrator's intended use for men becomes pretty much indisputable when noting that the illustrations in Dr. Granville's book on the invention of the electric vibrator exclusively feature physicians using it on men.

It is quite remarkable, then, that in just over one hundred years, our cultural perception has changed so drastically—from vibrators being designed specifically for men to an absolute taboo surrounding how men can use or benefit from them. It takes only a brief trip to an adult store to realize that nearly all vibratory products are specifically marketed to women—with bright pink shades, floral designs, and shapes like cute bunnies.

Without meaning to, I once worked in a high-end lingerie and sex-toy store. Now, that may sound like a phony excuse to tell the family, but it was true. The day after submitting my honors thesis, my best friend dragged me out for a shopping trip to cure my post-submission blues (it's a real thing!). During this trip—after consuming a couple of mid-shop champagnes—we found our way into this store, heading straight to the back, where we knew they'd keep the fun stuff. In between giggling and hitting each other with riding crops, I overheard two women trying to decipher how on earth a dual-vibration toy was meant to work.

With champagne confidence and an inability to keep fun facts to myself, I told them all about the history of the vibrator and its benefits. They ended up walking away with two each (pop off, queens), and the manager came to speak to us. She jokingly asked if I wanted a job. I, not so jokingly, accepted, realizing this was the perfect way to both fill the thesis-shaped hole in my life and put some of my niche knowledge to work. I started two days later.

I quickly learned that to get cis-male customers to purchase a toy you had to work extra hard. Selling the couples-compatible toy to heterosexual pairs shopping together was the gateway drug. After you had assessed whether you needed to dispel any stigmas of emasculation, the sell would be how the vibrator could not only enhance *her* stimulation during sex, but it could jointly be used during foreplay for *his*, too—a fact that generally took most men by surprise.

My time working in this store really brought home to me that our sex education had failed men as badly as it had the rest of us. Once or twice, men would return later (sans girlfriend or wife) and ask for clarification on where the different "pleasure zones" were on his body because he had genuinely never heard of them before. We laugh because so many men don't know how to locate a woman's G-spot, yet many men, as well as a lot of women, don't even know that their own P-spot exists. (For those curious, the P-spot refers to the prostate, possessed by people assigned male at birth. It can be stimulated internally and externally to create an intensely pleasurable sensation during orgasm. Internally, it's located about five centimeters inside the rectum; it can be externally stimulated by rubbing the strip of skin—the perineum—that runs between the scrotum and anus.)

Research into male vibrator use has been pretty limited; what exists is focused on heterosexual couples play. However, one study from 2009 found that the prevalence of vibrator use by men was surprisingly high. In fact, 44.8 percent of men studied stated they had used a vibrator during couples or solo play at least once (in comparison with 52.5 percent of women). Of those men, there was no significant statistical difference between those who identified as heterosexual, homosexual, or bisexual. Yet there was a notable difference in how these devices were used, with 91 percent of men stating that their use of a vibrator had occurred during sexual activities with women. While the number of men using vibrators may be high, it seems they are not using them on themselves—there still seems to be an existing stigma regarding men purchasing or using these products for solo play.

Our survey brought up similar results for men (though much higher numbers for others across the board). In the previous year, according to our participants, 73.7 percent had used a sex toy. Trans men were the highest percentage (79.1 percent), followed by trans women (78.6 percent) and then cis women (78.1 percent). Only 56.3 percent of cis men had pleasured themselves with the use of a bedroom aid, the lowest of any category. These numbers, though much higher than any previously recorded, still show a notable drop specifically for the male demographic. Why is this?

My guess would be that, as has happened with many commercial products throughout history, as soon as something becomes vaguely feminine in perceived use or marketing, the push to men completely disappears. In the case of the vibrator, once it left the physician's office and began its life as a household appliance, it was advertised as a domestic or medical item for the whole family. Looking over old advertisements from the 1950s, we can see women holding vibrators as though they were lipsticks. These pictures, decorated with cursive text, were proof that manufacturers were targeting the female consumer. See, it was the wife, after all, who placed the orders for the household. Miraculous claims were made: a vibrator could apparently cure everything from headaches and wrinkles to arthritis and tuberculosis. Not just that, this product was age-nondiscriminatory—an essential product for babies as well as a fantastic Christmas present for the grandparents (I would love to see how well that would go down now).

And, to reiterate, the one thing physicians such as Dr. Granville specified this prod-uct could not be used to cure was—all together now—*HYSTERIA!* In fact, even when vibrators were (in the more unusual case) used on women, physicians were advised to stay far away from any areas of titillating stimulation; as gynecologist James Craven Wood wrote in 1917, "the greatest objection to vibration thus applied is that in over-sensitive patients it is liable to cause sexual excitement. . . . If . . . kept well back from the clitoris, there is but little danger of causing such excitement." Even on these oc-casions when women were treated with the vibrator, there is far more evidence that they were undergoing this treatment to cure menstrual cramps than there is evidence (zero) of a cure for hysteria. The myth seems to have emerged from the coincidental timing of hysteria as a medical condition and the invention of the vibrator.

Why does all this matter? Because it matters how we tell history. In linking the story of hysteria and the vibrator, we achieve a story that is funny, cheeky, and a little bit sexy—perfect for Hollywood and Broadway adaptations. It's also insanely harmful. It paints women from recent history as mindless creatures who would allow doctors to essentially assault their bodies because their husbands said they'd been acting ir-rational. This isn't the story we should be telling.

So, how did the vibrator come to be the fun-loving bedtime companion of today? Well, for that you must thank your "ignorant, historical" woman. If Gosnell Duncan revolutionized the dildo, then our next dinner guest should be credited as Resurrector of the Vibrator.

Now, where on earth could Ms. Dodson be? What is that you say? She is running workshops in the drawing room? Gertrude Stein and Katharine Davis have gone to join her? Don't be alarmed, dear guest—Ms. Dodson's workshops are a safe and comfort-able space. I'm sure they will find her lessons quite insightful. Perhaps we should poke our heads in?

In the 1970s, activist Betty Dodson (1929–2020) created Bodysex workshops, which helped women learn about masturbation, their bodies, and empowerment through acts of self-pleasure. In these workshops, Dodson regularly employed use of Hitachi's now infamous product, the Magic Wand. Originally designed and sold as a back mas-sager, the Magic Wand was reborn in Dodson's skilled hands. Providing each woman with her own wand, Dodson taught her participants how to use the vibration and pressure to achieve vaginal and clitoral stimulation in a way that is most conducive to orgasm. This has become known as the Betty Dodson Method.

If enthusiastic reviews weren't enough, the success of this method has been determined by some fantastic studies. In 1979, the *Journal of Consulting and Clinical Psychology* analyzed the effects of different masturbation techniques on women who had difficulty climaxing, concluding that stimulation with the Magic Wand was most effective in solving this problem. More recently, in 2008, *The Scientific World Journal* published a research experiment that included five hundred women who previously struggled to achieve orgasm. Out of these, 93 percent found success using the Betty Dodson Method. Both objectively and subjectively, it can be concluded that this technique has game.

However, not everyone was as happy as these previously anorgasmic women about this wand's newfound magic. Hitachi was feeling quite the opposite. They continued to insist it was an innocent "personal care" item—but as their national sales manager at the time was to admit, "The people we hire know what it's for without us having to say it." Hitachi briefly stopped selling the device in 2000 due to concerns and conflict with their US-based distributor, though by 2002, it was back on the market—and it was selling *fast*. After featuring in an episode of *Sex and the City* (a moment of appreciation for our sex-positive queen Samantha), the Magic Wand completely sold out. Hitachi was far from grateful for this boost in sales; this, it seems, was one of the final straws. The company later discontinued this bestselling product due to concerns that its name would become attached to a toy intended for less-than-polite use. Yet its power was too strong to suppress. By 2014, production of the device had resumed, though Hitachi's name was dropped from its title. Thenceforth it was known solely as "the Magic Wand."

Betty Dodson's impact is not to be underestimated, and hers is a far better story than the one we've been told. Vibrators did not come about because doctors' hands were getting too sore from treating hysterical women. They have become the toy we know (and love) today because one woman took it upon herself to educate other women about how this simple household device could be wielded to achieve pleasure. It provided a solution to the problem identified by our friends Masters and Johnson—that the female orgasm is much more complex than we often presume it to be.

Most of the time, it takes a lot more than a penis in a vagina for women to achieve orgasm. Masters and Johnson called this the "phallic fantasy." Their report demonstrated that women's organismic pleasure was best harnessed by stimulating the clitoris, rather than with a thrusting member. Following this revelation, just over a decade later, Dodson came up with a solution—the Magic Wand, which could not only be used to stimulate the clitoris during solo play but also provide external stimulation while having sex with someone else. This opened women up to an entirely new world of pleasure—an experience of the body that is finally legitimized and recognized by research and education.

The Magic Wand and its imitators continue to be some of the bestselling sex toys today. In 2021, vibrators comprised 27 percent of the sex-toy market, while dildos were at 25 percent. In fact, I would go so far as to wager that this toy remains the most common gateway drug for many people into the world of buzzing bedfellows, finding a resurgence in sales particularly in the past few years.

(Self) Love in Lockdown

The use of sex toys has been on the rise for all genders over the past couple of decades: a general increase of nearly 10 percent between 2004 and 2014. (That's statistically significant!) However, this increase is very much eclipsed by the jump we have seen in the past few years. It wasn't just masks and sanitizer that experienced newfound popularity during the pandemic; sex-toy sales skyrocketed like never before. When online retailer Love the Sales compared their sales of adult toys in Australia from April 2019 to April 2020, they found a whopping 83 percent increase.

It wasn't just fluffy pink handcuffs, either—vibrators found their way for the first time into many nightstands. Adult-toy company We-Vibe claimed a 180 percent increase in sales to Australia from September 2020 to 2021; the women's sexual wellness brand Womanizer saw an increase of 200 percent.

Whether it was the absence of in-person dating, a consequence of finishing all of Netflix, or just general I'm-bored-in-a-house-and-I'm-in-a-house-bored vibes, the pandemic took us a long way toward normalizing bedroom toys. The effect doesn't just stop at the purchase itself; an increase in online purchases potentially means an increase in Google searches, an increase in views on educational content (good sex-toy manufacturing sites will generally include information on how and why to use their products), an increase in discussions surrounding use, etc. This all changes *and* reflects a change in our cultural responses to the use of sex toys. It's going to be interesting to revisit these statistics in a few years to see whether toy use dissipates once life returns to "normal" or whether sales continue on their upward trajectory. I predict it will be the latter.*

Of course, this normalization can hardly be said to be a unanimous attitude. You can almost hear the cries from the Facebook comments section—Are we going to let robots take all our jobs? This will be the death of human intimacy! However, those dissenters may be comforted to know the acceptance of bedroom aids is far from novel. Once again, there's nothing new today that we can't find in history, and we seem to be reclaiming the collaborative harmony in which we lived with such aids before—and I think it's safe to say we've managed to copulate just fine since. We have used sex toys to aid our sexual endeavors and we have used them to bury the dead. We have used them for fertility rituals and we have used them to add some extra spice into the bedroom. Sometimes they appear as sex *toys*, sometimes as sexual *aids*, and sometimes as a combination of both.

A good example of the latter is the cock ring (also known as a penile ring and constriction ring, but I, as always, prefer the crasser term). The cock ring's use in history was to both enhance pleasure (sex-toy territory) and to prolong an erection (sexual-aid territory). While its exact origins are uncertain, we can see examples scattered throughout history. The most commonly accepted origin is in the second Jin Dynasty in China (1115–1234 CE), and the design looked a lot different from how we may know cock rings today, as they were made out of the eyelids and eyelashes of goats. (I do hope you've finished eating!) The eyelid was first soaked and tied around the base of the penis. As it dried, it would tighten, helping the man stay hard for longer. The eyelashes were kept on for the extra stimulation they provided for both the man and woman. As strange as it may sound, this design still isn't entirely out of fashion—rings made of these animal parts can be bought online today.

Cock rings increased in popularity during the Song and Ming Dynasties. Thankfully, the design would go through a needed renovation. Similar to the dildos of the time, these versions were made of jade and ivory, designed to be slipped onto the penis before the man became hard. And, far anticipating the work of sexologists in the

* In 2021, revenues from the sex-toy market were $34.09 billion. Based on current trends, that sum is predicted to increase to $80.7 billion by 2030. Statistics sourced from Statista's sex-toys e-commerce report.

twentieth century, some of the ring designs would include a clitoral stimulator. One is a dragon wrapping around the ring and helpfully sticking out its tongue to increase the woman's pleasure.

This brings us to ben wa balls. Once again, their exact origin is debated, some believing they can be traced to the nineteenth century, while others place them as early as 500 CE. They were originally called *rin no tama*, translating to "revolving jewels" in English. They were two silver balls designed to be inserted into the vagina; one was hollow and one was filled with mercury (let's be thankful we've since updated the materials). Any kind of movement, be it walking, laughing, or swinging in a hammock, would cause these balls to vibrate and clash together—a rather pleasurable experience.

Rin no tama were adopted by sex workers in Japan, though it has been noted that they were also "well known by name to ordinary girls." Their popularity spread throughout Asia, finding a market in China and India as well. Anyone who has watched the Fifty Shades trilogy knows they are still popular today—and there is a good reason for it. They are exceptionally multifaceted in their benefits; for example, they enhance the impact of pelvic-floor-strengthening exercises. In fact, the health advantages are so well recognized that in Australia the purchase of ben wa balls can be covered by governmental health care. I would share this fact with anyone who would listen in my time selling sex toys, which made me realize how few people had ever heard of ben wa balls in the first place.

As well as the pelvic-floor benefits, ben wa walls can be a great toy for play, whether solo or mutual. Anastasia and Christian stans can testify to this. The pleasure they provide can be amplified by the movements from other partnered activities: be that spanking or anal or oral sex. The longer the balls are left in, the more aroused the wearer is likely to become, as the muscles contract around them. This pulsating generally continues in the moments after they have been removed, leading to an added sensation of tightness and pleasure for the penetrating partner.

It seems to me sexual toys and aids fulfill a fair few of our needs. They provide sexual *autonomy*—the ability to give ourselves pleasure without dependence upon another human. They are a source of *empowerment*—allowing people to both give and receive pleasure. And, of course, they give us *pleasure*—a pleasure that can be largely free from risks and complications, received through solo or mutual experience, and can be used to experiment with one's boundaries or to live within a delicious comfort zone. Sex toys have been with us since ancient times, before we even had any way to record their joys, and that kind of longevity truly deserves our respect.

I was working at the store one quiet day when an unassuming woman walked in. Realizing that nothing is more intimidating than a perky salesperson in a silent sex store, I hung around the back to assess if she needed anything. After a time of casual browsing, she gradually made her way to the back of the store to the sex-toy wall. *This is where I come in*, I thought.

"Let me know if you'd like me to explain anything to you."

Returning my polite smile, she continued scanning the wall. "That's OK. I just came in for one thing."

To my surprise, her search ended on one of the higher shelves. She reached up, then handed me a remote-controlled vibrating butt plug. "That's the last one," she declared matter-of-factly.

"What do you mean?"

"That's the last one—the last item from your store. I have the entire wall now."

I nearly dropped the remote-controlled vibrating butt plug. I needed to know everything about this woman *now*.

She was in her late fifties. Her entrance into the world of sex toys had begun little more than a year earlier—and she told me, without missing a beat, that it was one of the biggest regrets of her life.

"So many years wasted, because I was scared—but scared of what?"

Exiting a thirty-year marriage had finally given her the push she had needed to try something new. She had grown up in a conservative household, and for most of her life, the mere idea of sex toys was repulsive—it was what sad people needed to bring excitement to their marriages and deviant people needed for their perverted satisfaction; it was not what happy, normal people sought out. Only, she hadn't *been* happy. Until a year back, she had never had an orgasm. She had continued in a loveless marriage because it was "what you did." It was only after seeing her children grown up and thriving that she realized just how unsatisfied she was.

"My life all changed when I gave myself permission to experience pleasure. That is something no one should underestimate."

Pleasure is powerful. It is the driving force for so many things we do in life. Long gone are the days of Kellogg declaring a war on pleasurable food and activities. Pleasure is something we seek out, every single day, without even realizing it. Yet of all the ways we can experience pleasure, sexual pleasure is among the last to become normalized. I would like to think we are heading toward a time when, as it was for Diogenes, masturbation is on par with eating and shitting. When, as with these other bodily functions, we can have open and healthy conversations about what is safe and what is normal. Masturbation isn't going anywhere. Even after an entire war was waged against it, it was part of our lives. Women risked prosecution to make dildos for others, John Wilmot published poems in celebration of Signior Dildo, and Mrs. Phillips sold her wares and provided a safe space.

I think one of the reasons that our views on sex toys in particular have taken so long to renormalize is that they are caught in both our trepidation about sex and our anxiety about new technologies. The sex toys of today look very different (thankfully) from the siltstone dildos, mercury-filled balls, and goat eyelids of the past. Toys on the market now are body safe. They are rechargeable, remote operated, and sometimes even able to sync to an app on your smartphone. They really challenge our definition of sex. Are humans truly inferior to machines?

The answer, of course, is no; however, we need to recognize some of the limitations of the human body. Technology and other mechanical innovations are a large part of nearly every other aspect of our modern lives—so why not in the bedroom as well? I trust technology to do a lot of things I can't do and that benefit my life. In the same vein, I wouldn't expect my boyfriend's penis to vibrate with three different intensities and eight pattern settings. I have a vibrator that can do that for me—an item I know brings both pleasure and practicality into my life.

Toys also make sex more accessible, helping to improve sexual health, pleasure, and intimacy especially for aging and elderly people, those with disabilities or sensory disorders, and those limited by social or environmental constraints. They can provide a safe and fun way to explore one's own body and sexual desires for those with mobility impairments.

There's a real possibility to live in even greater collaborative harmony with sex toys. We have body-safe items on sale and the ability to spread good education about their benefits and uses. We also now have the opportunity to view masturbation, once again, as a normal bodily experience—with the added benefit of discussing why it should not take place in public forums (nudge nudge, wink wink, Diogenes). We've seen our views change considerably over the course of our history, and our unique position at this moment allows us to recognize masturbation as a normal part of being human while also looking to how technology can aid us in having safer and ever more pleasurable experiences.

QUEER KINKS

Let us retire into the library. There is no greater feeling than a full stomach, a good book, and some pleasant conversation.

Ah, look over there in the corner! I should have known I would find them all in here. The usual culprits—Woolf, Joyce, and Fitzgerald—have completely missed the soup! Shall we join them? Oh, they appear to be deep in conversation. Let us prick up our ears and see what droplets of wisdom we can catch.

"When I met him, Dr. Freud was sitting in a great library like this one, with little statues at a large scrupulously tidy shiny table. We were like patients on chairs. He was a screwed up, shrunk, very old man: with a monkey's light eyes, inarticulate: but alert."

Oh, dear. How lucky that Sigmund is still in the dining room. Come, sneak with me around the edges of the room—let's pretend we are looking for a book—and we'll see what else we can make of this talk.

"If you read Freud you know in ten minutes some facts—or at least some possibilities—which one's parents could not possibly have guessed for themselves."

Our poor parents' parents! (And our even poorer parents' parents' parents!) And to think Woolf is speaking to a world one hundred years ago! Today, Freud's theories do not need to be read and studied at length in the library—a simple Google search or quick YouTube may suffice to give us an understanding. What does that mean for our knowledge today? That really depends on the answer to another question.

"What does one know when one knows Freud? That knowing has *every-thing* to do with sex."

You have come to a halt (and just as their conversation was getting so juicy!)—what's the book that has caught your attention? Ah, the poems of Sappho! A personal favorite of mine as well. Let's give these three back their privacy and take our book to the coffee table to have a little read.

We have had a lively conversation about different sex acts and relationship structures that shape our sexual behavior. Now let us talk about what happens when sex and gender shape our social selves in even more all-encompassing ways—when they become a *sexuality* and a *gender identity*.

For anyone who has ever spent time studying history, the diversity of human sexuality and identity is impossible to deny. The liberalities of the ancient world pour off the page, with their concubines, cross-dressing romances, and gay orgies. But how did we move from these ancient liberalities to the persecution, prosecution, and even execution of gay people? If sexual and gender diversity is an immutable fact, where are the stories of these people throughout the centuries? And why does a general perception persist that queer sexualities and gender diversity are a "new thing"?

These are by no means easy questions to answer. But luckily for us, we have a while before entrées are served. Let's start by asking: Where were the gays and theys throughout history? Where were the trans men and trans women, pansexuals and asexuals, nonbinary and nonconforming people?

Well, the truth is, they didn't exist—but not in the way that "Karen Miller (proud dog mamma of four)" on Facebook would have you believe they didn't exist.

It is only in very recent history that we've begun categorizing these aspects of the human experience into a range of accessible labels. This doesn't mean they didn't exist—it just means we had yet to coin the names we know today.

When you learn the terms that were used before us, the experiences that have appeared lost to history begin to spill from the books. Rather than looking for "homosexual" or "gay," the ever-present history of queer people becomes far more obvious when we search the pages for "mollies," "sodomites," and "faeries." Equally, the diversity of gender experience is brought to the foreground when instead of "trans" and "nonbinary," we search for "hermaphrodites" and terminology that signifies a "third gender."

These stories have always been in the history books—we just need the right reading tools to be able to find them again. This is a task of great importance. We let those who have been underrepresented finally see themselves in the pages. We give lengthy and meaningful histories to the identities so many people today believe have none. This task of historical recuperation places us in a truly special position, though perhaps it means we're not quite as advanced as we think we are. As Fern Riddell has eloquently stated in her work *Sex: Lessons from History*:

Today, discussion surrounding gender or sexual fluidity is regarded as a unique moment in our sexual culture, when in reality it is closer to a return to the understanding of sex shared by our ancestors, albeit with modern protections in law to stop discrimination.

My favorite thing about libraries is that they make time travelers of us all. While we sit here in our cozy nook, we will allow our minds to travel between the present day, the late nineteenth century, the late twentieth century, and the ancient world, and then come back full circle. You'll hear the histories of some stigmatized and perhaps less understood identities, including bisexuality and asexuality. You'll meet some wonderful trans and gender-diverse historical figures.

Through this wide-ranging movement between subjects and historical periods, we'll come to better understand how queer people are at the forefront of creating labels to reflect our sexual and gender identity, but are also—perhaps paradoxically—leading the charge when it comes to redefining our identities as fluid and indefinable.

Which begs the question: Is there a contradiction between those two poles of thought, the notion of a fixed identity versus a fluid one? And if so, should we aim to resolve that contradiction, or should we let ourselves revel in these queer kinks?

Language and Labels

What's in a Name?

Queer: an umbrella term for people who are not heterosexual or cisgender (referring to a person whose gender identity aligns with the sex assigned to them at birth).

Outside the world of opposite-sex attraction, homosexuality and bisexuality are perhaps the most widely recognized "alternative" orientations.

Ah, do my ears deceive me? Who is that I hear coming through the front door? What a party we shall have now—Dr. Krafft-Ebing has arrived!

As you may observe, Dr. Krafft-Ebing's appearance is as eccentric as his views on human sexuality. His work has earned him a reputation as a most . . . shall we say, *colorful* character. But do not be alarmed, my dear friend, for while Dr. Krafft-Ebing's ideas may be considered risqué by some, they will illuminate our current conversation.

Homosexuality and bisexuality were first introduced in Richard von Krafft-Ebing's groundbreaking work, *Psychopathia Sexualis* (1886). *Bisexual* was from the work of a botanist, to refer to flowers that possess both male (pollen-producing) and female (seed-producing) parts. *Homosexual* derived from the Greek *homos*, meaning "same." Homosexuality had first been defined along with *heterosexuality* in 1869 by Karl Maria Kertbeny, though it would not be widely recognized until Krafft-Ebing's work.

This tipping point in the late nineteenth century—a little over 125 years ago—was the first time we felt the need to label and define various experiences of our sexuality and desire as a fixed social identity. But it's important to remember why these orientations and identities were defined in the first place. While thinkers such as Krafft-Ebing would advocate for tolerance toward people classified as "bisexual" and "homosexual," that was because these were classified as sexual "perversions" that deviated from "natural" sexuality—attraction to and desire for someone of the opposite sex. Krafft-Ebing believed this perverted sexuality to be a class of mental disorder.

In a very much no-win situation, Krafft-Ebing's work cannot find its place within either conservative or progressive ideologies today. Even at the time of its release, his work created immense conflict with religious leaders due to his recognition and proposed acceptance of sexual practices they considered sinful. By the same token, his work is unlikely to find any celebration within the contemporary queer community, as it advocates for tolerance on the basis of mental illness.

Regardless of its problematic basis, the immense impact of this tipping point cannot be ignored. The creation of terminology through which we can understand and consider sexual behavior as an identity, and allowing for *multiple* concepts of sexuality beyond opposite-sex couplings, was a foundation on which our more nuanced understanding of sexuality and orientation developed. Understanding how these terms came to be, however, is vital for understanding the discriminatory foundations the queer community was forced to build up from. It gives us a far greater appreciation for how these terms have been powerfully reclaimed today—and the work that was put in to get us to a point where they are used for education and empowerment, rather than to diagnose perversion and degeneracy.

When I first saw the statistics surrounding sexual identities in Australia, I can honestly say I was shocked. I had been turning to this study to help develop an argument about the prevalence of queer relationships in Australia—but I found myself utterly disappointed. In 2012 and 2013, the Australian Study of Health and Relationships published its research, which showed that only 1.9 percent of Australian men and 1.2 percent of women identified as homosexual. In even more stunningly low figures, only 1.3 percent of men and 2.2 percent of women identified as bisexual.

"Something has to be wrong with these statistics," I kept protesting to my mum. How many people were included in this study? Was it a diverse enough range of participants?* Had researcher bias skewed the results? On every front, I was made to see reason as Mum demonstrated the statistical validity. But seeing those low numbers seemed to clash with my own lived experience. I put it down in the end to perception bias, the small ways in which my life experience and the community I had amassed around me shaped the way I believed "everyone" saw the world.

So, should we just accept these figures? Are queer sexualities a tiny minority of our society, with everyone else engaging happily in heterosexual interactions for their whole lives?

Not quite. There was (thankfully) a point where the statistics began to contradict themselves.

If only 2 percent of Australian men (roughly 260,000) identified as homosexual, you would assume that roughly the same number of men would declare to have found themselves attracted to men or even stated they had engaged in homosexual relations. But when we look at these statistics, there is a significant difference between how people *identify*, whom they are *attracted* to, and how they sexually *behave*. While 97 percent of Australian men stated they identified as heterosexual, only 92.3 percent stated that they were *exclusively* attracted to the opposite sex. Even once we've subtracted the 1.3 percent who identified as bisexual, that is still a large number of men who have experienced homoerotic desire yet consider themselves heterosexual. These numbers rise again once we take behavior into account—of the population surveyed, only 90.7 percent of men had exclusively had sexual interactions with the opposite gender.

When we compare homoerotic *behavior* to homosexual *identification*, our numbers rise from around 3 percent to 10 percent. *That* is statistically significant—and something that certainly deserves critical attention. It was even noted in the study that for 4.4 percent of men and 9.5 percent of women, "sexual attraction does not match sexual experience." Similar data was obtained from the UK in the same year.

Now, of course an interaction with someone of the same sex does not necessarily mean you must ever after identify as queer (these statistics would skyrocket if we all

* We can see that, once again, the genders represented stubbornly adhere to a binary, and that a limited range of queer sexualities was accounted for. While this is definitely a point for improvement, it is unlikely it would have considerably skewed these numbers.

thought back to the games of spin the bottle in high school). However, it does invite us to raise the question of what goes into making the decision of our declared sexual identity—especially if it may be at odds with our past or present sexual behavior.

A decade after these studies, our survey similarly found a discrepancy between people's declared sexual identity and to whom they were attracted or having sexual experiences with—this time, however, the bridge between queer and heterosexual experience was reversed. While the majority of cis women were exclusively or predominantly *attracted* to cis men (61.1 percent), their sexual *experience* was exclusively or predominantly with cis men (80.6 percent). This is also true for nonbinary people. While only 19.3 percent claimed to be exclusively attracted to cis men, the majority of sexual experiences (46 percent) had taken place with cis men. It could well be that people are now choosing their sexual identities based on feelings of attraction, regardless of whether they have ever had any sexual experiences that match their attraction. This is a considerable ideological shift in the course of ten years.

Words matter. The meaning of these terms, how we have come to understand them, makes all the difference when it comes to these studies. At what stage are we given our QUEER membership card? Do we need to have desired a specific individual who was not of the opposite sex? How frequently do these desires need to have occurred? Do we need to have slept with this person? Are we officially queer only after we have had a queer romantic relationship? At what point are we gay, and at what point is it "just a phase"?

We all have entirely different ideas about what it means to be queer. This isn't necessarily something that needs to change. As we shall see, the fluidity of these terms and definitions can be one of the most powerful things about them. Words can flow and change as fluidly as our own desires. In another beautiful paradox, meaning emerges at the very point where there is no longer any need for meaning.

As wonderful and poetic as this all is, it does make it hard to study human sexuality. Reports on the prevalence of queer sexualities will continue to be skewed, confused, and contradictory when, as with the word *sex*, we don't have an established understanding of what these terms mean. Most recognize now that there can (and should) be steps taken by the researcher to suppress the confusion—such as a statement of how homosexuality and bisexuality are defined within the parameters of this study. But it also means that when we hear facts from these studies widely quoted ("If they're only 2 percent of our population, why do we spend so much of our goddamn time talking about them?"), they shouldn't always be taken at face value.

These numbers have a bigger story to tell, about the experiences, desires, and identities that have slipped through the cracks. The small contradictions to be found in these studies expose a larger search for meaning in our sexuality. I think that is a far more intriguing story to tell.

Speaking of stories, what is the book that our friends have pulled out? Still harping about Freud, I see. Let's have a listen to the essay they are reading . . .

> It is well known that at all times there have been, as there still are, human beings who can take as their sexual objects persons of either sex without the one trend interfering with the other. We call these people bisexual and accept the fact of their existence without wondering much at it.

Well, if we are to follow Freud's logic, it seems we can throw all these modern statistics out the window. One hundred percent of us are bisexual, and that is the end of that! While it was Krafft-Ebing who first used *bisexual* in terms of human pathology, it was our friend Freud who first used the term to describe desire. All people, in his view, were born bisexual—and would later evolve (kind of like Pokémon) into either homosexuals or heterosexuals. I choose you, Penis-chu!

Now, this may all sound like a whimsically queer utopia that conservatives fear the left want to incite. But the theory is a little bit more complicated than this—and it involves the desire to fuck your parents.

Ah, I am impressed we even got this far into the evening before bringing Oedipus into the situation. Would you be so kind as to bring that play down from the shelf?

Oedipus Rex is an Athenian tragedy written by Sophocles around the year 429 BCE. It has become best known as the basis for Freud's most famous theory—the Oedipus complex. The play begins with Oedipus, King of Thebes, investigating a plague that is ruining his city. He does what any good king would do and sets out to right the wrongs of his people—starting with a blind prophet, who tells him, "You yourself are the criminal you seek," and that Oedipus is the one who is truly blind. He tells Oedipus that he will one day be both husband and son to his own mother.

It transpires that Oedipus is in fact already married to—and sleeping with—his mom. Realizing the tragedy of the situation, he turns to the most logical solution—he decides to murder his wife/mother. However, a servant arrives with news: he is too late—Jocasta has hanged herself. In a state of madness, he takes the pins from her robes and gouges his eyes out—completing the prophecy that he would be the one who was blind.

Now, Freud must have read this play in his formative years, because he became absolutely *obsessed* with the predicament of Oedipus. He believed we were all a little like the tragic Greek king—didn't all of us want to fuck our mothers and kill our dads?

Freud's Oedipus complex is based on his other belief that all humans are born bisexual. As if one act of incestuous lusting simply wasn't enough, Freud believed we came into the world desiring both our mom and our dad. If an infant develops successfully in their early stage, they become a heterosexual. The male infant learns to repress his desire for his dad—becoming envious (and developing murderous intent) because Dad has a big penis and the baby doesn't—and continues lusting after his mom, growing up to look for a woman to replace her (Christian Grey, anyone?). If he is unsuccessful, the boy will become a homosexual, having mistakenly repressed the desire for his mom rather than that for his dad.* In all cases, bisexuality is eradicated, being a mere step on the way to the permanent homo or hetero islands.

Freud's work has been entirely disregarded by most (if not all) scientific communities. In 1996, the journal *Psychological Science* went as far as to publish a work that stated: "There is literally nothing to be said, scientifically or therapeutically, to the advantage of the entire Freudian system or any of its component dogmas."

Even still, it is possible to see how Freud's thinking and theories continue to creep around our world today—particularly in terms of bisexuality. While the belief that everyone is born bisexual is by no means widespread, his proposition that it is a "phase" on the way to a more legitimate sexual identity certainly took hold.

---

* Freud tried, unsuccessfully, to apply his Oedipal theory to women. However, like most of his interactions with female patients, it resulted in him rage-quitting and abandoning the attempt. He would forever curse the "riddle of femininity," describing women's sexuality as a "dark continent" that was near impossible to explore.

Orlando

A Bi-ography

While the term *bisexual* has been in use since the late nineteenth century, it is only in recent history that it has become broadly accepted and understood. It isn't only the straight mainstream that has endeavored to police the existence of various sexualities—this criticism has come from within the queer community itself.

There is, perhaps, no other sexuality that has been so heavily under the microscope for its political implications. In the latter half of the twentieth century, bisexual activism was met with strong resistance from many members of the lesbian community. For decades, lesbian and gay activists had worked to establish greater understanding and acceptance of the homosexual community. It's understandable how the "emergence" of bisexuality—describing a person who could experience romantic and sexual attraction to both men and women—could be perceived as a threat, undermining much of the work done to establish same-sex attraction as a legitimate experience. Between the 1970s and the 1990s, many lesbian activists condemned bisexual women in particular as opportunists, traitors, and political cowards.

The strength of the LGBTQIA+ community is undeniable. Its members have stood and continue to stand strong against oppressors through moments of horrendous tyranny. One of the reasons that it remains so strong is because of the solidarity many members feel with others in their community, even those they may not know personally. There is a shared experience, an expectation that other members will understand each other's struggles and hardships. But it is equally undeniable that initial resistance to bisexuality from many prominent members of this community delayed the broader social acceptance of this orientation.

In all my time at school (up until 2014), there was only one student who ever spoke about bisexuality. She would have been three or four year levels above my own, so I didn't know her well at all. However, the news that she had declared herself bisexual was so radical that it shook the school community. I was thirteen and I remember that she had a boyfriend when she came out, which made the whole thing so much more scandalous. I was watching them hug and kiss from across the auditorium as I eavesdropped on a conversation she was having in the meantime on what it meant to be bisexual, initiated by someone from my class who'd been dared to ask her. In what I now recognize as an incredibly articulate explanation, she said who she fell in love with had nothing to do with what someone looked like—it only had to do with how someone was inside. For that reason, she could find herself as attracted to girls at parties as she could to guys. I was absolutely mesmerized.

The dare-taker's verdict, however, was that she was a slut, and that was the attitude of the school at large. It was one of the last times before entering university that I heard bisexuality discussed in much detail—as a pseudo-identity adopted by girls who just wanted an excuse to make out with lots of people for attention.

In hindsight, that fact is not too surprising; out of my entire school, I believe we had one openly gay student and one openly lesbian teacher (whom other teachers instructed students to address only as "Ellen" for a bit of fun). It's fair to say it wasn't an inclusive environment, though of course we would discover it held *a lot* of sexually and gender-diverse people. Coming up to the landmark decade after graduating, I have watched so many of my previous peers come out as gay, lesbian, bisexual, transgender, nonbinary, and more. And while I welcome those posts and celebrate the joy old friends have in expressing themselves now, I also find it disheartening to know their self-acceptance could have happened much earlier.

The difference is, without a doubt, education. In our country Christian school, we did not grow up with an awareness of various sexual orientations and gender identities. You were the gender you were assigned at birth. You were attracted to the opposite sex—and the unfortunate, archetypical "gays" who did not fit that mold were the subject of bullying and harassment. I remember praying at night that I would not turn out gay—the worst thing I could imagine happening to me. We knew that some people were simply born gay, at least, so I would pray that wasn't me. I began praying around the age of twelve, when other girls first hung pictures of male celebrities in their bedrooms and lockers, excitedly talking about how hot they were. I didn't find any of them hot. After a while, I learned to fake the reaction the other girls were having. In a true low of adolescence, I would google "hot men celebrities." I still couldn't force myself to feel anything for them. I felt absolutely certain, in my gut, that something was wrong with me—and maybe, if I just prayed hard enough, it would heal.

Just over a year later, I would listen in awe to that girl from my school talk about bisexuality. That was also around the time I first watched *Buffy the Vampire Slayer.* I was instantly obsessed with Willow, the nerdy supportive best friend who dressed in atrociously patterned sweaters and fluffy hats. She was the first-ever media representation who clicked with me as relatable. And then I reached the fourth season. I was traveling around Australia with my family in the back of a caravan, watching *Buffy* intently on a portable DVD player. I finally reached *that* episode—a storyline that, at the time of its initial release in the early 2000s, made TV history. I watched Willow kiss a girl, and I felt something for the first time.

Now, as any good Slayerette will know, Willow had previously had a relationship with a boy (or rather, a werewolf). Still, the character would go on to depict one of the first same-sex relationships on television. This representation was groundbreaking for its time, and paved the way for so much more depiction and acceptance by mainstream media. With the position of hindsight, however, I see how this representation of *Buffy* also constituted bisexual erasure. At the moment she forms a romantic relationship with a woman, Willow is "gay now," as she reminds people multiple times throughout the remaining series. Even in one episode when, under the influence of a love spell, Willow falls in love with a man, this attraction is undercut by the fact she is "gay now."

There was no room for the fact that she had felt equally valid, and equally powerful, love for both a man and a woman during the series. One was her high school relationship, and one was her "real" identity. She was "gay now," and the love story from the previous seasons was rarely spoken of again. If *Buffy* were released today, I don't think this would be the story it would tell. Willow would have been a bisexual figure for young people like me to look up to and relate to.

The strange thing about my high school experience was that it was still acceptable to kiss girls. You couldn't date them (unless you were happy to accept what appeared to be a lifetime of Ellen-calling and ostracism), but you could kiss them. In fact, we kissed all the time. One of the things that most excited me about going to parties was the fact that you could kiss girls in games of truth or dare, albeit with the weird justification that we were doing it to turn the boys on. That made it OK.

I often wonder now how much of these years could have been spent in self-discovery rather than in a perpetual state of confusion, if there had just been better education surrounding sexual orientation and identity. Maybe the best friend I kissed that night could have begun exploring her bisexuality then, at fifteen, rather than at the age of twenty-six as a newly married adult. Maybe I would have saved myself many nights of praying—without understanding what I was praying for—to a god that I was in no way certain I believed in.

Even after that B was put into LGBTQIA+, politicization of this sexual orientation did not cease. One school of thought in radical feminism argued that bisexual women—given the choice of dating men and women—should swear off romantic involvement with the former. This was couched in the idea of being "better allies" to the queer and feminist movement—refusing further intimacy with cis men until issues of "toxic masculinity" had been resolved.

This line of thinking evolved from the idea of "political lesbianism," which originated in the second wave of the feminist movement of the 1960s. The concept was established with the publication of *Love Your Enemy? The Debate between Heterosexual Feminism and Political Lesbianism* (1981), cowritten by Professor Sheila Jeffreys and the Leeds Revolutionary Feminist Group. The book proposes that women stop engaging in heterosexual relationships as this serves patriarchal power—remove men "from your beds and your heads."

I remember this discourse about bisexuality circulating around the same time I was finally coming to terms with my own sexuality. Just as a concept of bisexuality had really been cemented in the minds of my peers, we now had the ideals of "good queer" and "bad queer" to contend with. This did little to improve mainstream perceptions of bisexuality. Even now, the reality of bisexuality is that we are defined by others according to whoever our partner is at any given time. In my times dating men, I was recognized as straight. I have regularly been asked if I feel guilty about being in a straight-passing relationship while identifying as part of the queer community. I think for many people, this feels like a having-your-cake-and-eating-it-too situation.

But my sexuality does not change depending on who I am dating or who I am sleeping with. Whether I am involved in a same-sex or opposite-sex romance, I am still bisexual. This means I have the capacity to both be sexually attracted to and romantically desire both men and women—and thus far, no interaction I've ever had has changed this. Bisexuality, by definition, refers to the capacity for sexual, romantic, or emotional attraction to two different genders (most generally, men and women).

In more recent times, this definition has been considered by some as outdated, as our idea of binary genders has changed with our idea of sexual orientation. This is the reason some people have decided to identify as pansexual instead—a sexuality that disregards gender identity—to explain their romantic and sexual attractions. This term encompasses attraction to men, women, nonbinary people, transgender people, and nonconforming people. It seems that just as soon as we have come to a relative acceptance of bisexuality, we have instantly outgrown the use of the label—a fact I believe we should be celebrating. It really shows how much faster we are evolving in our sense of education and understanding about sex and gender today than the world in which many of us grew up only yesterday.

It is likely because of this pace of cultural change that our survey showed a considerable rise in people identifying as nonheterosexual compared with previous surveys of comparable sizes. While 39.3 percent identified as heterosexual, nearly the same number identified as bisexual (33.8 percent). One factor of these higher results could be the fact they were collected via social media, largely from users interested in learning about sex education. However, this bias does not discount the number at large—many comparative reports have similarly collected their data through social media, but with very different results. It is far more likely that this rise is due to the recent movements and conversations that have helped to finally legitimize this sexual orientation.

It's this state of accelerating flux that makes it all the more pressing that we look back through the history books to discover how much things have changed, and how much they've stayed the same.

An Asexual History

B isexuality is far from the only identity that has increased in popularity. Homosexuality, occupying a space of around 2 percent in past studies, was reported in ours as 6.4 percent. While this number is deserving of attention in itself, one fact that really stands out is that nearly the same number of people identified as queer (6.2 percent)—and even more than homosexual was the number of people who reported their sexual identity as "other" (7.7 percent). This included a range of labels that were not laid out by our selected options, such as demisexual, pansexual, omnisexual, heteroflexible, panromantic, bi-polyqueer, polyamorous, abrosexual, polysexual, bi-curious, neptunic, fluid, questioning, graysexual, biromantic, demibiromantic, demiromantic, ace, omniromantic, ace bisexual, noetisexual, aroflux, aceflux, uranic, and sapphicbi.

This is an exceptional number of terms used to explain or define sexual orientation. A conservative person might look at this list and declare that sexual discourse has gone too far, when in reality, if we were to add the four categories of bisexual, homosexual, queer, and other together, these sexualities comprise well over half of our participants. This means that heterosexuality falls into the minority—the sexual orientation that has almost always dominated these kinds of studies.

What does this change mean? I think it's an indication that we are interrogating our sexual and romantic inclinations more closely than ever before—because now we have the terminology to do so. It is highly unlikely that most people would be familiar with the majority of these terms—nor do they necessarily need to be. What is important is that an understanding of them is available and accessible to those who are in the process of exploring their sexuality. Someone who finds themselves attracted to nonbinary and female genders can express their orientation as neptunic, or someone who can feel attraction only to those they are mentally connected to can explain this as being noetisexual.

These labels make communication of our desires and attractions easier for others to understand. Equally, discovering that there is a word for any aspect of our experience goes a long way toward legitimizing our attractions, allowing us to realize that they are indeed "normal" and shared. They can help us connect to others, creating a community for mutual education.

But it is only in the past half century that we have seen large-scale communities built around sexual identities—the concept of such identities, as we have seen, having emerged at the beginning of the twentieth century. These communities have been instrumental in creating belonging and acceptance for people who often felt deviant. They have been an invaluable space for education. I wonder if the riddle of historical figures categorized as having had a "complicated relationship with their sexuality" could be solved if they'd had this kind of language to express their experience.

Look! A new figure is joining us in the room. What an incredibly tall man! Did you happen to get a good look at his face? I can't quite make him out from here. What unseasonably warm clothing he's wearing—rugged up in his cravat and long coat, almost as if he doesn't want to be seen. It doesn't look as though he will be joining us; he is returning a leather journal to the writing table, securing it under lock and key.

Off he goes! Lucky for us, I happen to have a spare key. Should we take a little peek at what he left behind?

Of course! I should have known from that adorably awkward demeanor. Hans Christian Andersen (1805–1875) was one such "complicated" figure. Andersen was the author of such well-known fairy tales as "The Little Mermaid," "The Ugly Duckling," and "The Snow Queen." However, his personal diary (now in our prying hands) is far less suited to a Disney adaptation. Andersen kept a meticulous journal documenting each of his self-pleasuring sessions. On days he had enjoyed wrestling with his sea snake, he would mark the page with "++," sometimes providing some commentary about the experience. We have learned that it was not uncommon for Andersen to nip away in the middle of social gatherings to enjoy a little me-time. See here: "When they left, I had a double-sensuous ++."

No plus signs appear in the commentary tonight!

On the few days not marked with "++," Andersen would provide a helpful explanation as to why, such as "penis sore."

Despite his high libido, Andersen was deeply unnerved by the thought of sexual interaction with another human. One entry states that he was overcome with fear at the sight of a woman: "She stood there, half naked . . . I felt my whole body tremble" (January 6, 1834). In another instance, when his friend suggested that they find themselves some ladies, Andersen became so scared that he cried and ran away: "Two men came along and suggested women. No, No! I cried, and went home where I soaked my head" (February 28, 1834).

These interactions have led to speculation that Andersen may have been asexual. If so, he provides a fascinating historical point on the spectrum of sexuality. His lack of sexual interest in others does not prevent him from experiencing sexual pleasure himself, nor from forming romantic attachments. Indeed, it is highly likely that Andersen was biromantic, expressing desire for both men and women.

Now, in Andersen's time, ardent letters between men were commonplace. This was not an era of awkward half hugs between jocks and unexpressed bromance. Men of letters quite readily gave voice to the affection and love they felt for their close friends. (Honesty of emotions—what a radical idea!) Yet even by this standard, Andersen expressed a desire that went beyond the bounds of conventional friendship.

In one letter to his friend Edvard Collin, he writes: "I long for you, yes, this moment I long for you as if you were a lovely girl. . . . No one have I wanted to thrash as much as you . . . but neither has anyone been loved so much by me as you." In another: "I languish for you as for a pretty Calabrian wench . . . my sentiments for you are those of a woman. The femininity of my nature and our friendship must remain a mystery." Collin would write in his autobiography that he was unable to reciprocate the kind of love Andersen expressed, and was aware of the suffering this must have caused his dear friend. Yet, as the old wisdom goes, one must suffer to create art. Later, Andersen would not attend Collin's wedding. Instead, he would pen a tragic story to send to his friend—the story of a little mermaid.

Though Disney would Disneyfy the darker aspects of this tale, Andersen's preoccupation with an unrequited queer love is evident in the original work. This Ariel does not get a happy ending—she dies by suicide and her soul dissolves forever into sea-foam. In Andersen's world, humans are the only creatures with an immortal soul, while mermaids are doomed to live and die with the other creatures of the sea. When the little mermaid falls in love with the prince she has spied on, she makes a deal to become human—but the sea witch wants more than just her voice. As a condition, every step the mermaid takes on land will feel like shards of glass are penetrating her feet. Despite the pain, the mermaid must find a way to make the prince fall in love with her in order to keep her human form and immortal soul. However, his eyes are distracted by a beautiful woman, one who is truly human. The little mermaid watches in despair before diving one final time back into the sea.

> The little mermaid lifted her glorified eyes toward the sun, and felt them, for the first time, filling with tears. On the ship, in which she had left the prince, there was life and noise; she saw him and his beautiful bride searching for her; sorrowfully they gazed at the pearly foam, as if they knew she had thrown herself into the waves.

Perhaps if Andersen had had the terminology to express his romantic and sexual desires as precisely and openly as we can today, his stories would not have ended in hopeless tragedy. Perhaps he'd have realized that his aversion to sexual behavior did not mean his sexuality was dysfunctional, but that it was a sexuality in its own right—an understanding that has come about only within the past century.

One of the most common misconceptions about asexuality is that it describes the absence of sexuality—but it is simply another shape that sexuality can take. As early as 1896, Magnus Hirschfeld (a guest we shall soon meet!) made mention of people who experienced no sexual desire. It was also reported in Alfred Kinsey's research study in

1948, under the category of people who'd had "no socio-sexual contacts or reactions." Since its recognition as a sexual orientation, there has been considerable discrepancy among researchers in just how prevalent asexuality is, with estimates veering between 0.5 percent and 3.3 percent of the population. Our own survey lies in the middle, with 2.4 percent of participants identifying as asexual—though it's worth noting that this number may have been higher if we had not given participants the opportunity to define their own sexuality under the "other" category.

As our understanding of asexuality improves, we are recognizing how people experience it in a variety of ways. It wouldn't be entirely right to call it a spectrum, as there are multiple factors—such as sexual, emotional, and spiritual connections—that can inform one's experience of asexuality. Some people will experience no sexual attraction and no romantic interest in others; some will experience no sexual attraction but will experience romantic interest (suffixes such as *hetero-*, *bi-*, and *homo-* can be added to *asexual* to further define the multilayered orientation of an individual); some can experience sexual attraction only after an intense emotional connection has been formed (they might identify as demisexual); and others may sometimes engage in sexual behavior for bodily pleasure but feel little or no sexual attraction to others (graysexuality).

What is undeniably clear from modern research is the legitimacy of asexuality as an experience, orientation, and identity. And looking back through history, there are many more figures than Andersen who would likely have shared this experience. J. M. Barrie, the author of *Peter Pan*, is believed to never have consummated his marriage with his first wife, and was suspected by close acquaintances to not experience sexual desire: "I don't believe that Uncle Jim ever experienced what one might call 'a stirring in the undergrowth' for anyone—man, woman, or child. . . . He was an innocent— which is why he could write *Peter Pan*." George Bernard Shaw expressed to his friends that desire of the flesh held no interest for him. He would marry political activist Charlotte Payne-Townshend to avoid the scandal she otherwise would have endured living alone with him during his ill health. Charlotte was actively repulsed by the idea of sex, while Shaw remained uninterested until his death—that marriage, too, went unconsummated.

Codes and Symbols

Somewhere over the Rainbow

So we know that language can legitimize the experience of people belonging to sexual minorities, both for them and for how they are perceived by the wider world. But how can one word adequately convey the range of experiences of something as personal and subjective as sexual desire, behavior, and identity? And how have our uses for these labels shifted over time?

With Andersen's talent for hidden messages and codes, he could have been of great value to a community of his own. Throughout history, the queer community has adopted a range of code words and secret names to hide from prosecution and discrimination. Consider the adopted code "friend of Dorothy." Many may recognize this term only from unexplained references in pop culture: the Queen in *The Crown* (2020) rejecting a potential match for being "a friend of Dorothy," or, most iconically, when a character is described as "a disco-dancing, Oscar Wilde–reading, Streisand-ticket-holding friend of Dorothy" in *Clueless* (1995).

This term will be particularly familiar to older members of the LGBTQIA+ community. Calling oneself a "friend of Dorothy" was a secret way that queer people could identify one another in the first half of the twentieth century. Its usage was particularly prevalent during World War II, allowing men to safely identify one another. Before turning up the flirtatious vibes, someone could simply ask the other if they were a friend of Dorothy. If the answer was yes, especially if they were a *very* close friend, then it was safe to proceed. If the answer was met with confusion, the flirtation could be abandoned (rough luck if you were queer but out of touch with the slang of the day).

The exact origin of this slang is still unknown, though two candidates have been suggested. The first is in reference to Dorothy Parker (1893–1967). This Dorothy was an eccentric writer and socialite, married to a bisexual man (who described himself as "queer as a billy goat"), who frequently welcomed members of the queer community into her house. Another, perhaps more popular suggestion is in reference to *The Wizard of Oz*. Dorothy is played in this classic by the legendary Judy Garland, who became a powerful icon for the gay community. While Garland was not known to be queer herself, her personal struggles within Hollywood notably resonated with many people who felt like outsiders, during her lifetime and after. She was also closely connected to the queer community through family, as her dad, at least one of her husbands, and her son-in-law were gay. Her role in *The Wizard of Oz* has had lasting influences on the community. In fact, it is believed that the rainbow flag—the symbol of the LGBTQIA+ community—was in part inspired by Garland's rendition of "Over the Rainbow" in the film. The performance of Bert Lahr as the Cowardly Lion is considered camp, with the Lion referencing himself as a "sissy" (an effeminate term that was widely associated with the queer community). In the original writings of *Dorothy and the Wizard in Oz* by Lyman Frank Baum, he remarks: "Any friend of Dorothy must be our friend, as well."

By the late 1970s, the US Navy had discovered the shocking fact that there were many gay men within its ranks (a fact that should serve as a reminder of how far LGBTQIA+ activism has come in only fifty years). The undercover agents who were sent out to determine which of the troops were secretly gay caught wind of the fact that "Dorothy" was constantly referred to in their conversations. However, far from realizing this was coded slang, the Naval Investigative Service became convinced that a mysterious woman named Dorothy was a socialite ruling over the community of gay military personnel. A massive investigation was then launched to track down this Dorothy, in hopes that she could be coerced into revealing all the names of queer members within the navy's service. Unfortunately for them, this Dorothy was no more real than a singing scarecrow or a heartless tin man. While not many people continue to call themselves friends of Dorothy, there are other terms that, beginning as humble code names, have progressed to common language.

The word *gay*, for instance, meant "happy" less than one hundred years ago. So what happened? That question is going to take us to one modernist lesbian queen with a beautiful dancing dog named Baskets II (named after her first dog, Baskets I, died and she couldn't be bothered to learn a new name). But before we get there, we have to cover a little bit more history.

The word *gay* has been in use since the twelfth century, associated with being "joyous" and "brightly colored"; you could be in a gay mood or wear a lovely gay hat. It also took on wider meanings, such as elegant and stylish—perhaps because of all those brightly colored hats. It is because of this latter association with fashion that *gay* became associated with hedonism—a philosophical movement that promotes indulgence in pleasure, particularly bodily pleasures, above all else. By the eighteenth century, "gay house" was the name for brothels (I imagine because there were a lot of "happy endings" in these locations). Perhaps naturally for a practice that requires masterful oral skills, poetry was also called gay. In fact, the art of poetry was termed "the gay science," which informs the title of Nietzsche's philosophical work of 1882, to the amusement of many undergraduate students today.

Now it's time for our lesbian queen and dancing dog to drop onto the scene. Welcome to the library Gertrude Stein (1874–1946), the twentieth-century queer icon and prolific writer, who has been crowned "the mother of modernism."

Stein was a fierce and outspoken queer woman who lived openly on the Left Bank of Paris with her wife, Alice B. Toklas. She not only lived at the heart of the revolution— she *was* the revolution. Stein is an example of someone who, by doing something loudly and proudly enough, became unstoppable (#AlexanderHamilton vibes). She was a Jewish lesbian who refused to leave Nazi-occupied Paris, for crying out loud. Instead, she and her wife stayed to help get children out, care for soldiers, and protect the artworks of their friends. This would be an appropriate time to mention that their close friends, whose work hung on their dining-room walls, included Picasso, Matisse, Cézanne, and more—artists Stein practically discovered, and who are largely known today because of the efforts and risks she took to preserve their works.

It is believed that, in Stein's time, *gay* was used as a code word among queer people. In 1908, she started working on a short story called "Miss Furr and Miss Skeene." In this story, Stein takes all the various prior definitions of *gay*—happy, poetry, sexual promiscuity—and brings the coding to light, then gradually redefines it for the reader. For context, this five-page story uses the word a total of 140 times.

> *They stayed there and were gay there, not very gay there, just gay there. They were both gay there, they were regularly working there both of them cultivating their voices there, they were both gay there. Georgine Skeene was gay there and she was regular, regular in being gay, regular in not being gay, regular in being a gay one who was one not being gay longer than was needed to be one being quite a gay one. They were both gay then there and both working there then.*

Stein repeats and repeats the word *gay* in the context of these two women, until even the most oblivious of readers is likely to catch on that these women weren't just really "happy" together.

> *They were in a way both gay there where there were many cultivating something. They were both regular in being gay there. Helen Furr was gay there, she was gayer and gayer there and really she was just gay there, she was gayer and gayer there, that is to say she found ways of being gay there that she was using in being gay there. She was gay there, not gayer and gayer, just gay there, that is to say she was not gayer by using the things she found there that were gay things, she was gay there, always she was gay there.*
>
> *They were quite regularly gay there, Helen Furr and Georgine Skeene, they were regularly gay there where they were gay. They were very regularly gay.*

If there was ever a piece of literature to try reading out while drunk at a pub, I highly recommend this one. Stein's short story went to press in 1922. The *Oxford English Dictionary* credits it as the first use of *gay* meaning "homosexual"—we have the "mother of modernism" to thank for this one.

Oh, dear. Virginia Woolf doesn't seem too happy that Stein has entered the library. Look at her sneering across the room. Woolf never took a liking to her, thinking she was too convoluted, too repetitive, too *queer*. It is a good thing that Stein is engrossed in conversation with Magnus for now!

Of course, not all terms familiar to the queer community have kept their empowering and positive origins. Some have experienced the opposite journey.

Today, *transvestite* is widely considered offensive. This would probably surprise its inventor, Magnus Hirschfeld, an unforgettable icon in the story of transgender and queer advocacy. He was a gay Jewish cross-dressing sexologist, who became known as the "Einstein of Sex." Rather than devising a theory of relativity, he would open the Institute for Sexual Research in Berlin in 1919. By 1930, this institute would perform the first medically approved gender-correction surgery in the world.

At the time, this institute met with great success. Ideologies and movements that advocated for human tolerance and empathy were welcomed in Germany following the censorship it had seen throughout World War I. Hirschfeld advocated for the biological basis of sexual identity, as well as an understanding of "sexual intermediaries," the vast variety of people who fell in between the spectrum of "full man" and "full woman." He was instrumental in gathering six thousand signatures in a petition to decriminalize homosexuality in Germany (with signatures from some of our other dinner guests, Albert Einstein and Richard von Krafft-Ebing). Hirschfeld was also one of the first to bring to light the correlation of heightened suicide rates among the homosexual community and the prevalence of homophobic laws. By his estimation, at the start of the twentieth century, three out of a hundred gay men died by suicide each year in Germany, with a quarter attempting it at some stage in their lives. These facts—actual, tangible figures—changed the game when it came to the thinking about homosexual and transgender people. Naming the latter "transvestites" was an effort to legitimize, for one of the first times, transgenderism as a social identity.

Hirschfeld provided the medical documentation that enabled the performance of the first gender-correction surgery. Suffragist Karl M. Baer (born Martha Baer) would undergo this surgery in 1906. Baer was born intersex—an umbrella term covering people born with a variety of sex characteristics that don't fit typical binary notions of maleness or femaleness—and, as was and still is common, had been forced to present in line with a presumed gender throughout his early years. Hirschfeld's careful research would demonstrate that Karl was "in reality a man," and he averred that the lifelong sense of being in the wrong body had brought about constant suicidal ideation in Baer and taken an indescribable toll on his mental state. Baer's surgery was a success. He would go on to write a memoir of his experience by age twenty-two and was legally able to marry the woman he loved. Hirschfeld's institute would then become the site of the first male-to-female surgery as well as completing surgeries for many more patients. With cross-dressing illegal at the time in Berlin, Hirschfeld would also advocate successfully for passes for "transvestite" individuals to wear clothing of their affirmed sex in public.

In 1933, Hirschfeld's institute was attacked and vandalized by members of the Nazi party, who destroyed its extensive collection of books and artifacts. This was part of a broader campaign by the Nazis to suppress any ideas or information that did not align with their ideology, and many institutions and individuals in the fields of sexology and LGBTQIA+ rights were targeted. Hirschfeld fled Germany to escape persecution, and he died in exile in 1935. The destruction of the institute and the loss of its collection was a major setback for the field of sexology, and much of the research and knowledge gathered there was lost permanently. However, Hirschfeld's work and ideas had already had a significant impact on the way people thought about and understood sexuality—an impact that could not be lost to hatred and fire.

The influence of Hirschfeld's work was felt not only in Germany, but around the world. Many studies into the effects of homophobia and transphobia even today look back to his initial research. Though the term *tranny* was eventually adopted as a slur, rendering *transvestite* oppressive and degrading, even as recently as 1975, with the release of *The Rocky Horror Picture Show*, it was still untainted. When Tim Curry, the cross-dressing mad scientist, sang his iconic number, "Sweet Transvestite," it was intended as a celebration of transvestism, rather than the parodical performance some may consider it today.

A Tale of Two Sexes

People who today would likely be considered transgender existed, of course, long before it was given this modern name—and certainly long before the Sweet Transvestite from Transsexual, Transylvania. Excavated tombs and burial sites from all over the world have uncovered "perplexing" examples of men buried in the fashions of women and women buried in the fashions of men. One example that broke the media in 2011 was the skeleton of a "man" buried in Prague, estimated to be around five thousand years old. Men of this civilization were buried with weapons and their heads facing west, whereas this skeleton was found with its head facing east, surrounded by domestic jugs. This was highly unlikely to be a mistake. As archaeologist Kateřina Semrádová told *Czech Position*, "When a culture had strict burial rules they never made mistakes with these sorts of things. . . . We believe this is one of the earliest cases of what could be described as a 'transsexual' or 'third gender' grave in the Czech Republic." A 2018 study of the ancient burial sites at Teppe Hasanlu, Iran, estimated that 20 percent of the tombs did not conform to the woman/man binary. Artifacts found at the site depicted men in women's dress or engaged in the activities of women, as well as vice versa.

There are high-profile figures, even from ancient times, to whom we can look as early examples of transgender identities. The Roman emperor Elagabalus (204–222) is often regarded as one of the first transgender figures in history, and as perhaps the first person to look into the possibility of sex-confirmation surgery, as they offered vast sums to any surgeon who would be able to fashion them a vagina. It was recorded by the Roman historian Dio Cassius (c. 150–235) that Elagabalus would wear a variety of wigs and makeup, and request to be referred to alternatively as a lady, mistress, wife, and queen: "When Zoticus addressed the emperor as 'my lord,' Elagabalus responded, 'Don't call me lord, I am a lady.'"

Indeed, Elagabalus was far from the only famous Roman to challenge the boundaries of gender. Many consider Julius Caesar a gender-deviant figure, too. In some records of his life, Caesar is supposed to have regularly engaged in cross-dressing, even living as a girl in the court of King Nicomedes IV at the age of twenty. It was his long stay at this court in the first century BCE that set the ancient versions of the gossip tableaus alight, particularly because he was rumored to have committed the ancient sin of allowing himself to be penetrated during his rumored romantic liaison with King Nicomedes—Plutarch, a Greek historian, claims that Caesar served as a "queen" for Nicomedes. Following Caesar's victory in the Gallic Wars, Dio Cassius records that the people of Gaul allegedly comforted themselves by singing, "Caesar may have conquered the Gauls, but Nicomedes conquered Caesar." (A penis in the ass was apparently far more embarrassing than a Roman victory.) Suetonius (69–122), who was basically the Gossip Girl of ancient Rome, recorded more rumors that were spread about Caesar. With a reputation for rarely having his bed empty, he was described by his political opponents as *every woman's man and every man's woman*. The legendary Roman emperor, it appears, was truly indiscriminate when it came to love and mixed up in a series of sex scandals with both men and women, of high and low standing.

When taken at face value, the accounts of the time are clear—Caesar was a bisexual, active power bottom who made himself well known around many cities. But ancient history is a little bit more complicated than this. The accounts written by ancient historians were absolutely colored by bias and political motivation. Many of the accounts of Caesar's life were written well after his death, and often were wielded as a political weapon. In ancient Rome, accusations of same-sex liaisons were used to attack and discredit political opponents, regardless of whether these accusations held any truth. Today, some historians believe the relationship between Caesar and Nicomedes was a political fabrication, while others believe it's possible there was some relationship between the two men.

But what stories such as Caesar's can speak to—whether mere rumor or truth—is the close connection that has always been perceived between "deviant" gender identities and sexualities.

We can still see the complex ways in which gender and sexuality interweave. According to our survey, nearly half of trans women are more attracted to women (49.4 percent exclusively or predominantly)* and have more experience with women (39.5 percent exclusively or predominantly). The same in reverse is true for trans men. They are more attracted to men (38 percent exclusively or predominantly) and have more experience with men (37.5 percent exclusively or predominantly). Facts like this tend to confuse many people who are not too familiar with the trans community, as there is a common misconception of convoluting transgender with homosexuality. Remember that gender (such as identifying as man or woman) is different from sexuality (such as identifying as gay, lesbian, or bisexual). The assumption that transgender people must also be gay is a widely held misconception—even if statistics suggest that many enter into same-sex relationships.

There can be an abundance of reasons for this. Many transgender people end up in queer relationships because of the greater acceptance and understanding shown by the queer community. Dating as a transgender individual, even in the modern world, poses a variety of challenges. Many people who "pass" as cisgender have had to face a particular dating "etiquette" challenge: When is the appropriate time to disclose being transgender—or is there even a need to do so? If you do so up front, you may face immediate rejection, or worse, a threat to your physical safety. But those who have chosen not to mention the matter have just as frequently been met with hatred—accused of "catfishing" and "tricking" a partner into romantic or sexual feelings.

Both options open someone to hate crimes. While gender and sexuality are different, transphobia and homophobia often go hand in hand. The all-too-common scenario of cis men who find themselves attracted to trans women—and expressing anger or intention of harm upon discovering the other person to be trans—is a reaction that is rooted in a fear and hatred of homosexuality. If homosexuality were not equally

* The other 50.6 percent were divided between those equally attracted to men and women (28.4 percent) and those who were exclusively or predominantly attracted to men (19.8 percent). Finally, 2.5 percent were attracted to no one.

stigmatized, men wouldn't be concerned that they had potentially experienced homo-erotic desire. It is similarly rooted in the belief that trans women are not "real" women.

But this has not always been the case. In certain places and time periods, we have had far less trouble accepting transitioning gender experiences than we do today. Evidence of transgender people and their stories emerges in historical records. (Note that, throughout this chapter, I will refer to historical individuals with the pronoun of the gender they asked to be identified with, and not those they were assigned.)

François-Timoléon de Choisy, also known as the Abbé de Choisy (1644–1724), lived as a boy until fifteen and then as a girl until eighteen. They then dressed as a man for many years, before becoming known as a countess and working in the country to educate young ladies in the ways of polite society.

One 1932 publication reports on the AMAZING STORY OF GLASGOW WOMAN. LIVED AS MAN FOR MANY YEARS, positively reflecting on how this "woman" was joined in "marriage with another woman," had many male friends, and was described by them as "a fine little fellow."

All the way back in the 500s, we find the story of Anastasia the Patrician. A courtier to the Byzantine empress, Anastasia found themselves caught up in scandal as the emperor decided to romantically pursue them. As the empress turned jealous, Anastasia decided to flee from courtly life, running away from Constantinople. In Scetis they were granted protection in a monastery, moved into a cell in the middle of the desert, and thereafter lived the life of a hermit, as was permitted only to male monks. Anastasia dressed in the clothes of a man, practicing the life of a monk in near total seclusion for twenty-eight years. They continue to be regarded by many as a transgender saint.

Without a doubt, the stories of these individuals are scattered through the history books—and the best place to look for them is in past conceptions of a "third gender."

As passionate Facebook commenters will rarely let you forget, there are only two genders and that is the way it has always been. Pink is for girls and blue is for boys, and the Left Agenda is leading us to a giant gender-neutral-colored orgy. While the beliefs of Debra Whiller (good vibrations only ❤) and Patrick David (JESUS TAKE THE WHEEL) are far from correct, they do point at an interesting phenomenon in our cultural thinking. Especially in Western culture, the idea of a third gender category feels pretty novel. Yet many ancient cultures had a word for a third (and sometimes even fourth) gender category, which referred to experiences outside a gender binary: individuals who embodied both feminine and masculine qualities; individuals considered absent gendered qualities at all; or individuals who had both male and female genitalia. Nowadays, these identities would be better understood by conceptions of transgender, nonbinary, intersex, or nonconforming—modern terms that have roots back in the ancient world.

In ancient Mesopotamian mythology, there are many references to people who are not men and not women. A Sumerian myth references a being with no male or female organ. The sacred sex workers who acted in service to Inanna were described with reference to a third gender. These people played a key role in religious life and reportedly had the characteristics of both men and women—a concept that has proven a linguistic problem for researchers translating these texts into our modern binary language.

References to more than two genders also exist in ancient Indian culture. The Vedas (1500–500 BCE) describe individuals being assigned to one of three gender categories, described in the *Kama Sutra* as *pums-prakriti* (male nature), *stri-prakriti* (female nature), and *tritiya-prakriti* (third nature). The Hindu god Shiva is often represented with a dual male and female nature, and in Buddhist Vinaya, written in the early centuries of the first millennium, there are four gender categories laid out.

Similarly, in the premodern era (1258 through the eighteenth century), Muslim societies recognized five different manifestations of gender ambiguity: *khasi* (eunuch), *khuntha* (hermaphrodite/intersex), *hijra* (identifies as neither male nor female), the *mamsuh*, and the *mukhannath*. In classic Arabic, *mukhannathun* was a term used to describe people with ambiguous gender characteristics. Its definition evolved, variously referencing people who were lacking in sexual desire, effeminate, and later, homosexual. It is associated today with the "passive" male within homoerotic sexual encounters.

The Maya civilization is also believed to have recognized a third gender, describing both androgynous gods in mythology and divine healers of a third gender category in society. In the Inca civilization, individuals who occupied "a third space that negotiated between the masculine and the feminine" were vital to some ritual ceremonies, which at times included same-sex erotic interactions.

There are antecedents in the Western world, too. If *RuPaul's Drag Race* had been around, the Galli would have been hot contenders. They wore heavy makeup, bleached and crimped their hair, and adorned themselves in jewelry and brightly colored women's clothing. Despite online criticism that pronoun obsession is a sign of the world going mad, one of the most intriguing aspects about writings on the Galli is that their contemporaries changed their pronouns from "he" to "she" following their castration and initiation into the cult. "Poem 63" by Catullus describes the performance of this castration.

> *Then as he felt his limbs were left without their* man*hood, and the fresh-spill blood staining the soil, with bloodless hand she hastily took a tambour light to hold, you tambourine, Cybele, your initiate rite [emphasis added].*

Due to the classification of the Galli as women following their castration, scholars have felt rather confident in determining them to be an early example of transgender people. Others have thought that the Galli existed outside a dichotomy of male and female, and thus should be considered evidence of a "third gender." Both opinions have their merit. What we do know for sure is that the Galli provide an example of gender existing outside a strict binary in ancient Rome.

So why did these gender categories become lost to history? It's a consistent story having to do with colonization.

This was certainly true in Hawaii. Prior to colonial history, Māhū were a third-gendered people who occupied notable spiritual and social roles, such as priests and healers. They performed esteemed duties in the community and were considered exceptionally proficient in the care and education of children, as well as handing down cultural practices and stories. This was until Christian missionaries arrived in the first half of the nineteenth century. Because the missionaries could not conceive of a third gender, the Māhū people were considered shameful, effeminate men associated with same-sex interaction. Missionaries to Hawaii brought with them biblical teachings and anti-sodomy laws, and *Māhū* quickly transformed from a title of honor to a slur—a literal badge of shame, as many were required to wear a badge that marked them as their gender from birth. It took until the 1980s for *Māhū* to begin to be reclaimed by groups of queer activists, and now for some the term refers to various transgender experiences, while for others it harks back to a different notion of identity: teaching others, through expression of self, "the balance of female and male throughout creation."

A similar story is found with the Muxe people in the Zapotec cultures of southern Mexico. Today, Muxe people have been described as those "who appear to be predominantly male but display certain female characteristics," or alternatively, those who fill a "third-gender role between men and women, taking some of the characteristics of each." Once again, a third-gender system is reported to have been common prior to colonization of the area. The enforcement of Christian teaching brought discrimination that Muxe continue to face in many more Westernized areas. In spite of this, the Muxe community remains strong. Indeed, even in the early 1970s, it was estimated that 6 percent of the Isthmus Zapotec community were Muxe. As with Māhū of Hawaii, many artists, academics, and activists are continuing efforts to reinstate and remember these titles and the many stories they contain.

Gender Troubles

The Bluest Dress

As I said, the task of historical recuperation—finding historical figures who likely fit into our modern concepts of sexual and gender identities—is an important one, as it allows us to look at the long history of the words we use to describe ourselves. This project legitimizes; it makes us feel seen and heard; it makes us feel represented in a more solid, concrete way. History has a tremendous impact on what we consider "normal" today.

But when you look back through the archives, you also realize how unstable our foundations for gender and sexuality are. The ways we think about these concepts are themselves fluid, and constantly in flux at different moments in history—and even within individuals themselves.

One of the stories I believe truly highlight the ambiguity of gender definition is the fervor with which we have adopted the tall tale of *blue for boys, pink for girls*. Before the mid-eighteenth century, all babies were dressed in white cotton dresses. This was a far more logical solution for the ease of changing diapers, not to mention the ease with which dirty garments could be bleached. The same cannot be said of brightly colored dinosaur onesies (if you know, you know). Clothing was gender neutral until children reached the age of six or seven—only at the turn of the twentieth century did pastel colors became a fashion fad; however, not in the way that we know them today.

Pink was linked to masculinity, and blue was linked with femininity. From the *Earnshaw's Infants' Department* trade publication of 1918:

> *The generally accepted rule is pink for the boys, and blue for the girls. The reason is that pink, being a more decided and stronger color, is more suitable for the boy, while blue, which is more delicate and dainty, is prettier for the girl.*

This was the accepted rule in department stores until the 1940s. What happened then is still debated. At the same time, many countries saw the rise of "the New Woman," the stereotypical figure of a "masculine" woman who was educated, fought for her career, perhaps worked in traditionally male fields as a result of World War II, and took part in radical activities such as bike riding and pants wearing. Retailers would have likely been under pressure to keep up with these progressive times and the widespread interest this figure sparked (which, concurrently, could spark a nice financial boost). There is a possibility that retailers began marketing pink clothing to women as a result, as the New Woman was depicted in the masculine pink color. If this is the case, it is even more laughable that today such conservative ideals have become attached to this color dichotomy.

There's a more unfortunate possibility, too. During World War II, in many concentration camps, the pink triangle was used as an identifier of gay men, meaning "effeminate" qualities were also associated with pink. This symbol has since been reclaimed by the wider LGBTQIA+ community to protest homophobia and as a marker of resilience.

Our widespread indoctrination of *blue for boys, pink for girls* shows how truly arbitrary our thinking about gender is. (I mean, how many wildfires* are we prepared to risk for an ideal that is not even a century old?) It also reflects the ebbs and flows of history. We aren't always moving in one direction toward progressive ideals and liberation. During World War II, the New Woman came to the fore, and then, as we

---

* The El Dorado wildfire in California, which started on September 5, 2020, was caused by a smoke-generating pyrotechnic device at a gender-reveal party. The device, which was intended to release either blue or pink smoke to reveal the gender of the baby, instead sparked a wildfire that went on to burn more than 22,000 acres of land, destroy homes, and cause the evacuation of thousands of people. The couple who hosted the party were charged with involuntary manslaughter and other offenses.

moved into the 1950s, we saw the conservative Stepford Wife ideal. We can regress as well as progress.

Stories like these also demonstrate how connected our understanding of gender is to our understanding of sexuality. In this instance, the policing of "gendered clothing" in the eighteenth century sought to achieve an eradication of homosexual desire (a desire that, prior to that moment, had not even been given a name). As historian Randolph Trumbach has summarized:

> *What the nineteenth century called homosexuality and heterosexuality are not distinctions to be found in universal human nature. They were, instead, products of a gender system that had appeared in the early eighteenth century and that accompanied the new forms of marital friendship and paternal affection.*

In the early years of the eighteenth century, at the onset of the Enlightenment, the definitions of what it meant to be a man and woman were shifting. Policing of gender and sexuality took on a practical reality. Children, who were initially socialized together for the early formative years, were now stridently separated. Clothing became a powerful weapon. Boys were sent away to schools to be educated in entirely male spheres, and were dressed in breeches to mark themselves as separate from the tainted world of femininity. For women, this entailed a stress upon more romantic ideals of marriage and of the sacred duty of motherhood.

Intriguingly, prior to this century, women were regarded as the more sexually charged. They were generally represented as having an unruly, all-powerful sexual desire—which is the reason they needed the more constrained man to keep them in their place. This all changed come the Enlightenment. "Women were not whores." They were now demure creatures, intended for a life of domesticity, who engaged in sexual activities only for the purposes of producing a family. For men, this ideological change largely centered on a distancing from effeminacy. Masculinity became defined as the absence of homoerotic desire, a force that naturally turned man's attention away from his procreative purpose. As a result, the act of sodomy became increasingly stigmatized and more severely prosecuted. This ideological change was politically motivated: an effort to place more stress upon the structure and importance of the perfect family—a cultural priority that continues to affect us into the modern day.

Before this ideological shift, homoeroticism played a rather prominent role in European life. The work of Trumbach has gone a long way in bringing this side of history to light.

> In Europe before 1700, adult men had sexual relations with both women and adolescent males. Only relations with women in marriage were legal and approved of by the church. But men engaged in other relations with women, ranging from prostitution to adultery.... Sexual relations between two males were similarly illegal, immoral and yet honorable when conducted in ways that displayed adult male power. In most of Europe and certainly in England, this was achieved when adult males sexually penetrated adolescent boys.... These sexual relations between men and boys did not—and this is the essential point—carry with them the storage of effeminacy or of inappropriate male behavior, as they began to do after 1700 and have continued to ever since in modern Western societies.

This kind of relationship is a form of pederasty—a dynamic that is thankfully and rightfully shunned today. Pederasty is often discussed now as a perverted practice from the ancient world, ignoring the fact that it was practiced in Europe until as late as the eighteenth century. Looking back to such cultural practices can help us to understand how vastly our concepts of "appropriate" sexual desire and behavior have changed over time.

In ancient Greece, pederasty was a homoerotic relationship between an adult man (erastes) and pubescent boy (eromenos). This practice was undertaken by society's elite, marking an important transition of the young man into his career as an adult. It was the responsibility of the erastes to educate and provide guidance to the eromenos. Education was intimately linked with homoerotic love—the erastes could provide adequate social training for his eromenos only if he loved him deeply. There were strict rules surrounding the erotic relationship that the two were allowed to engage in, centering on a distinction between physical love (eros) and nonsexual love (philia). The boy could not demonstrate any sexual love toward his mentor. Doing so would have been considered a sign of weakness, deeming him "womanlike" for his desire to be penetrated. The only sexual relationship allowed between the two was intercrural sex, taking place between the boy's thighs, along with other signs of affection. Failure to show these signs of affection toward young boys was taken as an insult, as illustrated in one moment from Aristophanes's play *Birds*:

> A fine thing there between you and my son,
> you old spark. You met him coming back
> from the gymnasium, after his bath—
> you didn't kiss or greet him with a hug,
> or even try tickling his testicles—
> yet you're a friend of mine, his father.

We can all be grateful that this piece of the past has been left behind.

The ancient Greeks even had a god of homosexual love, called Ganymede. Little to no concern was given to the gender of the person one desired—all that mattered was who was on the top and who was on the bottom. As Paul Chrystal has summarized, "What was important was not that one practiced sodomy; it was *how* one did it." Allowing oneself to be penetrated carried the same stigma as performing oral sex; these acts were a sign of weakness and effeminacy. This didn't mean there was any shortage of butt stuff—in fact, "Greek love" referred to the act of anal sex due to its prevalence across Greek cities. Upperclassmen could engage in anal sex with men lower in the social hierarchy, such as enslaved people or sex workers—in this form, homoerotic behavior was encouraged for, and even expected of, Greek citizens.

Similar conceptions of anal sex existed in ancient Egypt. As archaeologist Charlotte Booth remarked, identifying homosexuality in ancient Egypt is "a difficult task . . . because the concept of homosexuality, as we understand it, did not exist in the ancient

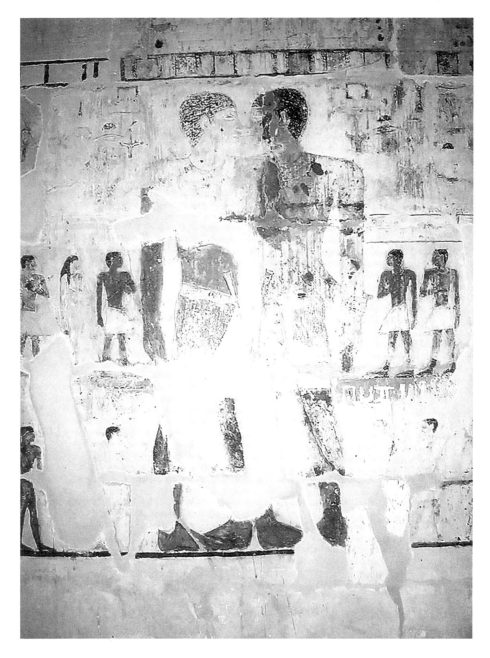

The depiction of Khnumhotep and Niankhkhnum from the outer hall of their shared tomb. Niankhkhnum stands on the left, while Khnumhotep is on the right, with his right arm affectionately placed on Niankhkhnum's shoulder.

past." Same-sex relationships were categorized in ancient Egypt according to who was penetrated and who was penetrating. *Nkkw* or *Hmiw* was the term given to the man who was penetrated, which carried connotations of effeminacy and cowardice. This didn't so much carry homophobic connotations—as there was no stigma attached to being the one who was penetrating—as it did misogynistic ones.

Khnumhotep and Niankhkhnum are often described as the first homosexual couple in recorded history. This belief is largely based on a depiction of two men standing nose-to-nose that decorates the shared tomb of these two "royal confidants"—the manicurists of the king. It was considered a highly revered position, as the role required daily proximity to the king. This image, while appearing innocent today, was the closest artwork would get in ancient Egypt to depicting a kiss, as portraits of the deceased had to have unobscured profiles in order for their spirits to regain their bodies in the afterlife. This kind of saucy position was usually reserved for married couples. The tomb also features depictions of men holding hands and embracing, thus unsettling historians' favorite explanation that they were brothers or just really good friends. In other illustrations in the tomb, Khnumhotep adopts positions that would have been considered "feminine," such as smelling lotuses, leading scholars to suggest he is depicted as the "wife."

Both of these men were recorded as having wives and children, family members who were likely also buried in the tomb. While their wives are both depicted, neither is in anything close to the positions of intimacy shared by the men. Intriguingly, there appears to be evidence of attempts to erase the wives from various drawings in the tomb, but it's unclear when this defacement took place.

Metamorphoses

n the past, research has focused on finding a biological basis for our sexual orientations. Researchers are now looking into the ways these can change throughout our lives. One study from 2015 explores new ways of conceptualizing sexual selves, desires, and relationships outside the traditional categories of heterosexual and homosexual. Researchers referred to the more overlooked statements of the likes of Alfred Kinsey, who once found that "very few people are exclusively homosexual or exclusively heterosexual; instead, most people fall at other points along the continuum." It was their determination that sexual orientation is fluid and can shift over time:

> *An individual's orientation might be heterosexual at one point in life, bisexual at another point, gay at another point, and heterosexual again at yet another point. The existence of multiple orientations at different points in the life of course does not mean that an orientation at a particular point is "truer" or more "real" than an orientation that exists at another point.*

It seems Dr. Freud's belief that we are all bisexual, while entirely misinformed, is also strangely on the right track!

The researchers of this study claimed their qualitative data reveal the new ways people are beginning to "shape and redefine their sexual selves outside of traditional normative categories." It is understandable that many members of the queer community may push back against claims such as this. The idea that sexual orientation can change over time could be seen as contrary to the legitimizing identities this community has worked so hard to define. Moreover, it may also invoke the insidious practice of "conversion therapy"—the pseudoscientific process of changing someone's sexual identity, often through intrusive and traumatizing means. I believe, though, that rather than undoing the work of LGBTQIA+ activists, this line of thinking opens a liberating way of thinking about sexuality.

As we've seen throughout our time in the library, our categories of sexual orientation—such as homo, hetero, bi, pan, and so on—are created and determined by society. They function well as tools for helping us understand both ourselves and others, as well as finding empowerment within a sense of sexual identity. Nevertheless, no human is limited to a single definition. Our sexuality, our sense of self, is far more powerful than this, and capable of evolution.

Perhaps we would be wise to recall the more fluid conception of sexuality that was common in the ancient world. As classicist Eva Cantarella has remarked in reference to ancient Greece:

> *Homosexuality was not an exclusive choice. Loving another man was not an option out of the norm, different, somehow deviant. It was just a part of a life experience; it was the show of an either sentimental or sexual drive that, over a lifetime, alternated and was associated (sometimes at the very same time) with love for a woman.*

Changes in one's situation and environment could equally affect one's sexual behavior. It has been speculated by historians that the reason Spartan women began to cut their hair short was so they could look more like their husbands when they returned from war. Homosexuality was as common in Sparta as it was elsewhere in ancient Greece—during their time away in battle, men would "come together" to boost morale. Accordingly, women perhaps kept their hair short to make sexual relations more familiar for their husbands when they returned home.

Women were well regarded in the city of Sparta. Unlike girls in other city-states of ancient Greece, who would finish their education as young as thirteen, Spartan women were expected to stay in school until the age of twenty, the same age as their male peers. It was only after this time that proposals for marriage could be considered. Once married, the woman became the master of the household above her husband. With the men away at battle for unpredictable periods of time, it made perfect sense for the women to be in charge. They took care of the finances, the agriculture, and the operation of the home, and had the final say in any decision regarding their properties. And, just as the men kept each other company on the battlefields, relationships between women were fairly standard.

Women were not only equals in education and intellectual discussion but also regarded with the same amount of respect. Spartan men who died on the battlefield and Spartan women who died in childbirth were honored with the same mark of respect— their names inscribed on headstones near the city, having died as heroes.

Another figure whose sexuality may well have fluctuated over time was Sappho of Lesbos (630–570 BCE), renowned philosopher and poet from ancient Greece. On the island of Lesbos, Sappho ran a community that educated women and girls. Homoerotic relations were a big part of education, experienced both between the girls in attendance and between students and teachers. As homosexual love played a massive role in the conception of masculinity and community for ancient Greek men, Sappho believed the same should go for women. While most of her poetry has been lost to time (only "Ode to Aphrodite" remains in its complete form), her words about homosexual love between women continue to resonate with many today.

> *And her light*
> *stretches over salt sea*
> *equally and flowerdeep fields.*
> *And the beautiful dew is poured out*
> *and roses bloom and frail*
> *chervil and flowering sweetclover.*

Prior to the nineteenth century, *lesbian* referred to anything that had come from the island of Lesbos. This included wine. (Save me a bottle of Lesbian wine, please.) This changed by the end of the century to refer to "a kind of love that used to be practiced in Lesbos" (wink wink, nudge nudge), though Aristotle was referring to fellatio as "lesbi-azein" even back in ancient Greece because it was so commonly practiced on Lesbos.

Despite her incredible writings and philosophies, Sappho was dismissed by her contemporaries because "she is a woman" and remembered by historians as a "sex-mad little whore." Despite the bad press during and after her time, Sappho's legacy continues. She is depicted in Raphael's work within the Stanza della Segnatura of the Vatican (right across from the famous *School of Athens*) as the "tenth muse" of ancient Greece. Though she is largely remembered as a queer icon, it is highly likely she was married to the man with whom she had her daughter, Cleis. One of the most famous stories about Sappho is that she jumped to her death from a cliff because of her love for a ferryman. Some scholars have claimed that this was done in an effort to heterosexu-alize her (which, as we have seen from history, is a likely story). If it was true, however, then Sappho could serve as an example of someone with fluid sexuality.

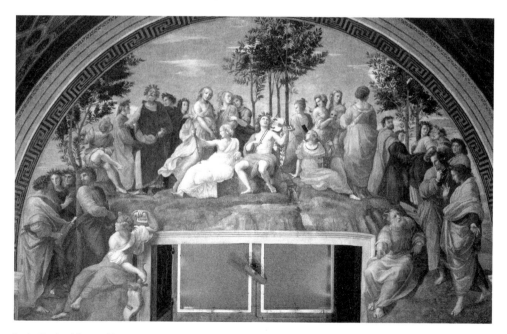

In the Raphael Rooms (Stanze di Raffaello) in the Vatican Palace, Rome, lies *The Parnassus*, a fresco by Raphael created between 1509 and 1511. In the bottom left-hand corner of the masterpiece, the poet Sappho is elegantly portrayed, holding a scroll with her name inscribed upon it.

"I've been drunk for about a week now, and I thought it might sober me up to sit in the library," Fitzgerald is explaining to Stein as she inserts herself into their group, to the obvious disdain of Woolf.

"Fitzgerald," Stein announces, ignoring her friend, "has written a book for the New Generation. He will be read when many of his contemporaries are forgotten." She now fixes her inexorable attention on the scrawny man on her other side. "Joyce is good. He is a good writer. But who came first, Gertrude Stein or James Joyce? Do not forget that my first great book was published long before *Ulysses*. But Joyce has done something. His influence, however, is local. He has had his day."

"I hate intellectual women," Joyce mutters in retort, his pride clearly suffering under the unapologetic declarations of Gertrude Stein.

Stein's booming voice must have reached the dining room. Look, as everyone gathers to hear what she has to say! Here come Hemingway and Picasso, Matisse and Henry James. Have you ever seen anybody so quickly take command of a room?

Woolf has clearly had enough of the conversation. With a pointed roll of her eyes, she has picked herself up and . . . Oh, it seems she is making her way over here!

"Look at them," Woolf sneers, exerting no effort to hide her contempt of the growing crowd. "All gathered in honor of Miss Gertrude Stein, who is throned over there on that broken settee. This resolute old lady is inflicting great damage on the New Generation. She keeps insisting that she is not only the most intelligible, but also the most popular of all living writers!"

"I may say," Gertrude Stein's voice rings across the room, "that only three times in my life have I met a genius and each time a bell within me rang and I was not mistaken. . . . The three geniuses of whom I wish to speak are Gertrude Stein, Pablo Picasso and Alfred Whitehead."

With a loud and frustrated sigh, Woolf storms out of the room.

It is truly a shame that Woolf and Stein were never able to resolve their differences, considering how much the two had in common. Both women helped to lead the modernist art movement, heralding in, as they called it, the *New Generation* of writers and readers. Both women were proudly and openly engaged in romantic relationships with other women, becoming queer icons.

Perhaps we should tell them how greatly indebted we are to their bravery, how the love letters Woolf wrote to Vita Sackville-West have been read over and over by so many of us as we explored our sexuality; how Gertrude's small, graffitied phrase *Gertrice/ Altrude*, scribbled in the margins of one of her manuscripts before she handed it to Alice to edit, is a reminder to always be loudly proud of the people you love. Those small moments of history, which perhaps meant little to them at the time, have had a significant impact on so many who came after. I think they ought to know.

If one thing is certain about *our* new generation, it is that the number of queer people is on the rise. Even back in 2014, from the small percentage of men who identified as queer on the Australian national survey, the majority came from a younger age bracket of sixteen to twenty-nine years old—33 percent of men identifying as homosexual and 27 percent identifying as bisexual. In the 2022 Gallup poll, 7.1 percent of respondents said they identified as LGBTQIA+, 86.3 percent said they were heterosexual, and 6.6 percent did not offer an opinion. LGBTQIA+ identification doubled from 2012. The largest demographic of people we identified as queer came from Generation Z—a grand total of one in five people. Millennials were the next biggest age demographic, at 10.5 percent (with bisexual being the most common category).

This can tell us a lot about how cultural perceptions of sexuality have changed in very recent history—really in the blink of an eye, compared with the histories we've been tracing. This younger age bracket had increased access to education and awareness of various sexual identities—and it's "perfectly queer" this can go a long way in improving your understanding of yourself. New ways that people connect have opened a possibility to change this conversation. We are in a truly unique position, with immediate access to information as we have never had before—and we are undeniably seeing the effects.

One thing that also needs to be considered is that older generations may still be reluctant to identify as queer, due to prevailing fears of repercussions. This reasoning was voiced as such by researchers working on a study that produced similar findings.

One of the most important findings of this study is the higher proportion of younger people reporting as a minority sexual identity. This suggests that a cohort effect may be at work. Sexual identities and the willingness to disclose one's identity can be influenced by the social attitudes and legal environment of the time when each cohort passes through their formative years. Older cohorts have spent much of their lives during a time when social acceptance was lower than it is today, and this might still influence how some of them report their identities.

Continued discourse on gender, sexuality, and identity is imperative if we want to keep ourselves from slipping back into a time of increased intolerance and discrimination. Of all our changing stances and opinions, nothing encapsulates humans' complete indecisiveness better than our continually changing stance on these topics. We simply cannot decide if we love these topics or hate them, if we should politely choose to ignore them or do nothing but speak all about them. We have flip-flopped, pivoted, and done 360-degree backflips so repeatedly throughout history that it is a genuine challenge to identify the dominant stance at any moment. From where we sit today, however, it is a bit easier to see that queer sexualities and identities are experiencing a widening acceptance and celebration, though we still have a long way to go.

As we speed, therefore, toward another tipping point, we should pause to consider the queer possibilities of the future, based on what we have learned from the past. We have seen times when sexuality was considered an indefinable and fluid part of ourselves, and times when it became a marker for persecution and diagnosis, and our present moment, in which we are increasingly forthright about our sexual and gender identities.

How does the world we have created today speak to those moments of the past? Will we continue to be as fascinated by labels and language to capture identity? Will we interrogate new forms of fluidity—more of a focus on desires and behaviors than a set identity—which, it could be argued, is a return to an ancient mindset? Perhaps the solution is found in the combination. Sexual identity can continue to be a source of empowerment and community, while we recognize that focusing too much on a set identity may close us off to different desires and behaviors. History is a cyclical, ever-moving beast—what new direction can we imagine for ourselves before the wheels turn again?

Speaking of moving, it is time we should go. Best to defuse the growing tension between Woolf and Stein. There is no better solution to all problems than a good game shared with friends. Let a round of festivities begin!

THE KINK KINK

The time has come for festivities and games. What do you say? Shall we join the others in a little play before dessert? Joyce and Fitzgerald have hidden themselves somewhere in the library. (How wonderful that Joyce's wife, Nora, has finally joined us—and just look! She has brought along their cats.) Freud and Krafft-Ebing are inseparable, engaged in a heated debate about perversion and normality. Out come Jean-Jacques Rousseau and C. S. Lewis, Theresa Berkley and Philostratus—there are still so many figures with whom we can become acquainted!

What activities are on the table for us tonight? Take a tour with me through each room, and let the fun begin.

Role-play, spanking, foot worshipping, and electrostimulation. Kinks and fetishes are a distinctly human phenomenon. As Dr. Kate Lister adeptly expressed, "While all animals have courtship rituals, no wildebeest has ever gone into therapy because it's struggling to express a latex fetish." As far as I know, we have so far been unsuccessful in finding another species that gets off on the sight of a leather-clad dominatrix torturing their testicles or the touch of a pedicured foot. Depictions of our more freakish proclivities have hovered in our peripheral vision for years. Think of the leather-clad gimp who featured, unexplained, in one memorable scene in Quentin Tarantino's *Pulp Fiction* (1994). Or the famed placement of Margot Robbie's stiletto heels on Leonardo DiCaprio's face in *The Wolf of Wall Street* (2013).

We are all aware that some people enjoy more than your traditional hanky-panky. What I don't think many of us know, however, is just how prevalent these "alternative" desires are. It isn't just a mere few who enjoy things a little freakier. In fact, recent research into the prevalence of fetishes consistently concludes that half (if not more) of respondents report some kind of kinky desire. A 2017 study of the Belgian population found that 46.8 percent of participants had performed at least one BDSM-related activity, with an additional 22 percent stating they had fantasized about it. These activities and fantasies would be classified as "kinky"—the acronym BDSM standing for bondage-discipline, dominance-submission, and sadomasochism. Only a year after this study, a similar finding emerged from Czechia, which reported that 51.1 percent of men and 39.4 percent of women (45.9 percent of all respondents) were sexually aroused by a dominant or submissive partner. By that account, more of us than just Leo would enjoy getting a stiletto to the face.

What I find so shocking about this number is not necessarily how high it is (there are, as we shall soon see, more than enough kinks and fetishes to go around), but the relative silence on the topic. If one person in every two is fantasizing about being spanked, whipped, collared, and dominated, it is genuinely mind-blowing that these topics remain so deeply shrouded in shame and secrecy. Who decided that licking someone's genitals was normal behavior but straying down to their toes was a no-go? And if we have, as a collective, agreed to this unspoken rule, why do these desires refuse to go away?

The internet! I can almost hear the storms again of those angry Facebook commenters. *The media is to blame! MTV! TikTok! It was Britney Spears in that darn red latex catsuit!*

Let us pause for a moment before we begin the festivities. This is sure to be the most *interesting* part of the night thus far. We are going to alight on everything from BDSM and role-play to cuckolds and chastity belts. We'll visit twentieth-century America, medieval China, ancient Mesopotamia, and early modern Europe.

Through it all, we'll come to understand a few significant things about kink. By definition, kinks and fetishes are viewed as aberrations, far less often discussed and more stigmatized than other sexual practices. For this reason, it remains acceptable to "kink-shame" in a way that other forms of social shaming are no longer permitted in progressive circles. To many, kink remains shrouded in silence and secrecy.

And that is a shame indeed (pun intended), because kinks and fetishes can present us with a chance to explore the most richly surprising, boundary-pushing aspects of human sexuality. Kink radically destabilizes received wisdom about the purpose of sex. It's about expanding our *erotic* life rather than a purely sexual one. Kink is about experimenting; it's an imaginative and even emotive practice. Within boundaries that are reciprocal, consensual, and respectful, kink can be a way to explore real-world dynamics, particularly relating to power and gender. And above all, it can be a hell of a lot of fun.

We are, in our contemporary moment, starting the work to shake off persistent stigmas, and part of that project involves looking back to, well, kinky history (who could have guessed?). Despite what your disgruntled aunt might declare at Christmas, the dominance of these "perverted" desires can hardly be blamed upon the rise of the digital world. Long before people were buying the bathwater of their favorite internet gamer girls, they were buying the sweat of their favorite gladiators in ancient Rome. Long before hentai pornography rose to prominence, people were admiring erotic tentacle art in seventeenth-century Japan. And long before that pesky internet could bring us raunchy emails, James Joyce was penning love letters about his wife's beautiful, fragrant farts and excrement.

Of Humans' Bondage

Joyce, it really is a pleasure to join you again this evening. I'm so glad your wife could make it. If I could just move your cat, we will join you for a game.

In 1957, James Joyce's letters were sold to Cornell University, securing a small fortune for his family. In 1975, a selection was published by biographer Richard Ellmann*—and it's fair to say they blew people away. In the world of Joycean scholarship, they are referred to simply as "the dirty letters"—or, as I prefer to call them, "the fart letters." The fart letters exposed not only an intense love for his wife, Nora Barnacle, but also a reverence for the talents of her backside.

> *You had an arse full of farts that night, darling, and I fucked them out of you, big fat fellows, long windy ones, quick little merry cracks and a lot of tiny little naughty farties ending in a long gush from your hole. [December 8, 1909]*

Joyce's hope that "Nora will let off no end of her farts in my face so that I may know their smell" was far from a one-time fancy. Indeed, this was a common theme.

> *Fuck me if you can squatting in the closet, with your clothes up, grunting like a young sow doing her dung, and a big fat dirty snaking thing coming slowly out of your backside. [December 16, 1909]*

---

* An edition that is now out of print—however, many of the letters were published online and preserved.

The letters penned to his lovingly named "sweet naughty little fuckbird" regularly circulate through internet forums and university corridors. It only took until my first week of studying Joyce as an undergraduate for one student to dramatically perform (slam-poetry style) a selection of their favorite lines before the tutor arrived.

> *I wish I could hear your lips spluttering those heavenly exciting filthy words, see your mouth making dirty sounds and noises, feel your body wriggling under me, hear and smell the dirty fat girlish farts going pop pop out of your pretty bare girlish bum and fuck fuck fuck fuck my naughty little hot fuckbird's cunt for ever. [December 9, 1909]*

Yet, despite popular demand (including the desperate pleas of many undergraduate students), Nora the fuckbird's responses to these letters have never been released. No one is sure what has happened to them—my guess is relatives kept them a secret after seeing the memes created out of Joyce's side of the correspondence. Whatever Nora wrote to excite Joyce to such a point of filthy euphoria has been left to our dirtiest imaginations.

> *Goodnight, my little farting Nora, my dirty little fuckbird! There is one lovely word, darling, you have underlined to make me pull myself off better. Write me more about that and yourself, sweetly, dirtier, dirtier. [December 8, 1909]*

It is entirely understandable that many serious Joycean scholars physically shift and twist in discomfort at the mention of "the dirty letters." That discomfort, I believe, boils down to two reasons: first, these letters made a laughingstock out of an otherwise serious and prolific writer; and second, even celebrated figures deserve to have a private life that remains just that. It can be hard to impart the profound cultural significance of Joyce's work when the class is reading "pull up your dress a moment and hold [the letters] in under your dear little farting bum." Yet, I think there is something significant that the circulation of these letters adds to our perception of Joyce, and by extension, any "great figure" in history: they, too, are human.

The fact that the Great Figures of History enjoyed sex—let alone kinky sex—is still shocking to us. I personally think it is something to celebrate that the author of *Ulysses* (1920)—a book that is considered the modernist bible, that experimented so artfully with the limits of writing that it practically rewrote the rules of literature itself—is the same person who found bliss in hearing and smelling "the dirty fat girlish farts going pop pop" out of his wife's "pretty bare girlish bum." How much more could we learn from the past if we stopped erasing the sexy, kinky bits? We could understand a lot more about what it means to be human if we talked about these parts of who we are, who we have always been, and stopped clouding them in shame. If Joyce, who embraced the sexual satisfaction he found in the desires others may consider freaky, still found his way onto the coveted list of Great Figures of History, what on earth is stopping us from doing the same?

Though we don't have Nora's replies, there is a lot we can tell about her, and their relationship, from this one-sided correspondence. From the "lovely word" that Nora underlined to the topics Joyce implores her to "write more about," we can see a relationship and sexual desire being mutually, respectfully explored by two loving and consenting parties. What they're doing (once, I suppose, you remove lines such as the desire to lick Nora "like a ravenous dog until [her] cunt is a mass of slime") is actually rather beautiful.

At this time in their relationship, Joyce had traveled to Dublin while Nora was left with their two children in Trieste, Italy. Instead of allowing this absence to suspend their desire for each other, the two turned to pornographic letters. And what is more, Nora initiated it. Around November 28, Nora must have written a dispatch that Joyce had longed to receive—"A letter for my eyes only." Whatever Nora wrote, it was enough to inspire a string of filthy correspondence that has remained a shock even after a hundred years.

As the writer Brenda Maddox noted in an article in *The Guardian*, this is no small feat for a Galway girl who had attended school for only a few years at the Convent of Mercy. As you may know personally from underwhelming sexting attempts, there is an art to writing that really gets the blood boiling. Eggplant and peach emojis aren't going to cut it on their own. Nora must have had the literary talent, as well as intimate knowledge of her receiver, to write the perfect sexy letter—a letter that inspired a man known prior to that for avoiding obscenities to keep up with the style of his "little cuntie."

With depictions of women's sexuality so scarcely recorded in history, this correspondence should stand as a celebrated example of a sexually empowered figure—one who not only initiated this infamous discourse, but is also recorded to have slid her hand inside Joyce's trousers on their first date in Dublin in 1904. In many ways, Joyce and Nora provide a wonderful example of how sexting or phone sex might still take place in an ethical and respectable way. They experiment with the bounds of a sexual fantasy and mutually experience pleasure; Nora encouraged to "Tickle [her] little cockney" and Joyce assuring her that he will "lie down and pull at [him]self till" he comes.

How different is this from the online sex many of us had during the pandemic? Wouldn't it have been wonderful if instead of believing we were the first to experience this sort of encounter, we could have looked to a historical couple whose written legacy demonstrates ethical, respectable, and loving experimentation? It goes without saying that the pandemic affected many of our sex lives—in fact, an argument could be made that it encouraged many to explore their kinky boundaries and interests. Similar to those cuddle parties that followed the influenza pandemic of the past century, the COVID-19 lockdowns and border closures inspired us to explore human touch and connection in new ways. Clearly, the combination of this health crisis and the technological advancements of recent years provided the perfect environment.

Many lovers started locking each other down, too. Out of all the adult products that skyrocketed for retailer Love the Sales in 2020, bondage toys—such as handcuffs and restraints—experienced the starkest rise. Australia became the number one country searching for these products on this site, with a whopping 125 percent increase over previous years. As someone who experienced it firsthand, there must be a correlation with the fact that Melbourne had the longest lockdown in the world. (There are only so many puzzles to do, OK?)

It wasn't just Down Under that was doing it dirtier. A study looking at sexual behavior during the pandemic in the USA, UK, Australia, Canada, and more reported that one in five people were mixing up their sex lives, and there was a strong correlation between an improved sex life and those who had decided to spice things up in the bedroom (nonetheless, 43.5 percent of people reported that the quality of their sex lives had declined). Those who had decided to use the pandemic to experiment tried new sexual positions, acting out fantasies, role-play, and even BDSM.

Pandemic-related experimentation was not just limited to those lucky enough to lock down with a sexual partner or partners; people explored a range of BDSM-related activities and fantasies within a virtual space as well. In 2020, when kink and fetish dating app KinkD put out a survey to 3,495 of its users, it found that virtual BDSM play topped the list of sexual activities during lockdown: the top ten in order included virtual sex (using technological communication to arouse each other or mutually masturbate), dominance-submission play, orgasm control (purposefully denying, forcing, or extending someone's orgasm), bondage, anal play, age-play (role-playing as a different age), foot fetish, role-play, voyeurism (watching someone in a state of undress or when engaged in sexual activity), and sadism-masochism.

According to the cofounder of the app, John Martinuk, the online world places no boundaries on participating: "Unlike real-life play, cyber play allows you to indulge in the Dom/Sub scene or relationship merely through technological means, with no face to face communication." For some people, this freedom from a face-to-face aspect is taken literally—you can have a virtual BDSM relationship without ever revealing your face. Dominance and submission relationships in the virtual world include sending erotic messages and instructions, sending pictures or videos, and participating in live video chats.

An example of this was explored (though in the form of sex work rather than dating) in the popular first season of *Euphoria*, which went to air in 2019. One character, Kat, becomes a virtual dominatrix, with her identity hidden behind a cat mask. Over video calls and text messages, Kat instructs her submissives when they are allowed to touch themselves throughout the day, when they are allowed to orgasm, and when they need to send her money (financial domination). The latter being a kink I will *happily* help anyone out with if they would like my bank details.

For many people in real life, the virtual world is preferred when it comes to exploring kink and fetish play. Anonymity can provide a new level of confidence to set boundaries and take risks, perhaps even to speak to others about desires people may otherwise feel embarrassed to confess.

Erotic Charges

One of the primary reasons that these explorations translate well into the online world is that, in contrast to popular belief, kinks and fetishes don't have to have anything to do with sex. Kink identity and experience can be physical, emotional, spiritual, and mental. One recent study determined that while sex often overlaps into the experience, kink generally has more to do with intense physical sensations (like sadomasochistic play) or power exchange. One participant, described as a thirty-two-year-old white pansexual transgender female, stated, "Kink is more important than sex to me—kink is more erotic to me than anything else." This is an important distinction. When is kink sexual and when is it erotic? And how can kink—a concept so culturally synonymous with sex—ever be removed from sexual desire?

While there is plenty of overlap, eroticism is distinct from a sexual experience. Eroticism can be an experience of arousal or sexual excitement that isn't linked to the desire to have sex. You could see a painting in your local gallery of a half-naked woman and recognize that it is *erotically* charged. The painting may arouse your imagination and emotions, but that doesn't necessarily mean you have any desire to fuck that painting. That is one surefire way to get yourself banned from the Louvre.

It is this desire or intention toward the sex act that really distinguishes something that it is "sexual" from something that is "erotic." In the case of this respondent, it is the *erotic* feelings—such as arousal of the imagination, exciting physical sensations, playing with power dynamics—that she prioritizes in her experiences with kink above actually having sex.

As kink can be removed from sex, it is also suited to being a solo activity, whether or not it's considered sexual and erotic. As a fifty-year-old bisexual cis male from the same study described:

> *I would, with leather gloves on, bind my hands with rope and suspend myself by wrists quite often to masturbate. Never touching myself—just from the tightness of the rope and the leather gloves. I would hold myself up off the floor so I could smell the leather on my hands and then I would cum.*

Or this forty-seven-year-old bisexual cisgender female:

> *I would do things like take straight pins and put them in my boob or my butt. Spank myself, just crazy shit.*

Even when BDSM practices do involve other people, it is common to find that the erotics of the experience will be prioritized above factors that would generally be considered central to sexual desire. For instance, gender often has little to no bearing when it comes to selecting a partner for BDSM play. Practitioners report prioritizing personal connection over gender. As well as this, compatibility in one's preferred BDSM role was given more weight when making a choice about a romantic, sexual, or play partner: for example, finding a partner who wants to take control if you prefer being more submissive, or finding someone who enjoys the sensation of pain if you enjoy inflicting it. Really, this is just a matter of practicality—I can't think of anything less productive than two submissives lying there, waiting for something to happen.

The limited weight given to gender in many BDSM practices perhaps explains its popularity with nonbinary and nonconforming people. Of the 36.5 percent of our participants who said they had engaged in BDSM-related activities over the previous twelve months, the highest demographic was nonbinary/nonconforming people, with half saying they had taken part (48.9 percent). In fact, these activities were more popular with gender-diverse participants than with those who were cisgender. Trans men were close behind (47.7 percent), followed by trans women (42.5 percent) and those who described their gender as "other" (41.4 percent). Cis women were not too far below this (36.1 percent), and cis men made up the lowest demographic (32 percent).

Now, none of these numbers can be construed as low—the statistics speak to the popularity of the practice across the board. However, it is interesting that our cultural representations of BDSM are often rooted in heteronormativity when this is far from the case. It is hard to divorce cultural perceptions of dominance and submission from an image of a powerful businessman in suit and tie, and the clumsy and relatable brunette he falls in love with. (If you haven't watched *Secretary* [2002], this is your sign to do so.)

Indeed, this perception even slips into our sexual fantasies. A study done by the Burnet Institute, in Melbourne, found that 70 percent of its participants enjoyed watching porn in which men were portrayed as dominant; this was the second most popular category of pornography. Yet the world of BDSM—those who practice it knowingly in communities and those who perhaps unwittingly dabble in related activities in their bedrooms—is so much richer than this.

My first experience with the kink world was virtual. I was playing *Second Life* at far too young an age, and unwittingly stumbled upon the reason the game has an age restriction. This game allows you to create an avatar and explore the multiplayer virtual world. I was on the phone with a friend, giggling our heads off after we had dressed our avatars in outlandish costumes and explored a user-created city. Suddenly, we saw a crowd of other avatars also dressed in bizarre costumes. Some were wearing tails and cat ears, others nurse and teacher costumes. There was even a group dressed as riding instructors—my friend was a massive fan of the series *The Saddle Club*.

A costume party! We were so excited. With a click of our mouses, we teleported ourselves into the party.

The party hall wasn't quite what we were expecting. We'd entered a red dungeon filled with cages and decorated with chains. Most of the avatars were no longer wearing their costumes. We lowered our voices to whispers over the landline phone, fearing that our parents might be able to hear what we were doing. We had no idea *what* we had stumbled on, but we knew we were not meant to be there. Between snickers, my friend suggested that we should click on a free object nearby, just to see what would happen.

"No way!" I wheezed. "You have to do it first!"

"Let's do it together," she suggested, seeing the item was suggested for two users. "On the count of three?"

After what felt like the longest countdown of my life—in between giggles and *oh-my-god-no-ways*—we finally clicked the object. All attempts at being quiet were thwarted. We burst into hysterical laughter, as our avatars suddenly stripped and began hitting each other with riding crops.

We teleported out of that world *fast*.

For my first experience with an actual kink club, in my early twenties, there were still the costumes, there were still the cages and the chains, and there were still nervous giggles. Shortly after I had begun working in a sex store, I decided to go to an event to write an article, following the advice of a friend, who suggested I couldn't just hide behind a computer screen and research papers—I needed to see the scene firsthand. I dragged her along for support; there was no way I was going into it alone.

"Where are you folks off to tonight?"

"Just a club," we both mutter, looking anywhere but at each other.

The driver nods and says no more.

He doesn't notice the collar around her neck or the crop underneath my leather skirt. We try our hardest to conceal our laughter—we're a $55.45 Uber away from cementing ourselves as kinksters.

We're among the first to arrive at the hired club, having clearly missed the memo that late is sexy. The place has been decorated like an underground dungeon, filled with cages, crucifixes, and suspension devices, which equally excite and terrify me. My first order of business is to find the bar.

"Excuse me, are you up for auction tonight?"

A middle-aged man, clad in nothing but latex booty shorts and a harness, addresses us from a respectful distance. I watch his gaze rise from my friend's leather pants to her collar, following its chain into my hands.

"Oh, I'm sorry." His attention falls on me. "Will *you* be putting your slave up for auction tonight?"

I stare at him blankly, unsure whether I should be laughing or driving a hard bargain. My friend looks equally conflicted. Giving the collar a little tug, I attempt my best impression of Christian Grey. "She's not for sale, sorry."

We find that the collar offers us immunity as we explore further, leaving us free to sip our G&Ts and watch spankings undisturbed. I take on the role of tour guide, explaining to my friend what's happening as people are suspended with rope from the ceiling and covered with suction cups on tables.

Most displays we move past quickly; others have us mesmerized. We watch an experienced submissive and dominant for the longest time. The submissive is on her knees before the dominant, transported into a state of ecstasy with each lash from his whip. He is nurturing her, loving her.

By the time of the auction that everyone keeps mentioning, we're tipsy. We follow the crowd up five twisted stairways. We have no idea what's happening, but we're excited. We're still pretending we're only here to gain creative inspiration, to grow as artists. We don't discuss my tightening grip on her chain.

The rooftop is at capacity. We find a bench at the back and watch as a wild variety of people are marched onto the stage. Gimps, adult babies, Venus in Furs, fluffy dog costumes. They're all offering various services for fluctuating prices.

We're swept up in the excitement. We're shouting and cheering, throwing around fake money, helping neighbors secure their prizes. A submissive with vibrating underwear is currently at the podium. The women behind us have just been overtaken in the bidding. I gather some fallen money from the floor.

A dark-haired woman hesitates before accepting it. "Can you be up for auction instead?"

I laugh, deflecting.

"I mean it."

Her words send shivers straight down my spine.

The crowd dissipates quickly after, as lucky purchasers guide their slaves to darkened corners in the building. I check for my phone and wallet. I ask if my friend is ready to leave.

"I kind of want to *do* something." She's looking at me, pleadingly. I'm shaken, but I say I'll stand by and watch.

We make our way back down the stairway, listening to the echoes of slaps and shouting. It's coming from the second floor. Curiosity leads us into the gathered crowd. A woman is straddling a spanking horse, her arms and legs tied to each of its wooden legs. Two dominatrices are at work, smacking her, caressing her cheek, stroking her hair only to pull it.

Just as they finish, I realize they're the women who were sitting behind us. The crowd cheers as their subject is helped from the horse, expressing her gratitude to the two mistresses. That's when they see us. The leather-clad dominatrix walks confidently up to my friend. She looks at me for approval and I hand over the chain. Before she takes my friend away, she says to me, "Why don't we try it together?" But I don't move.

My friend is secured onto the horse. I watch as they prepare her, adjusting the restraints, asking about her tolerance for pain.

Suddenly, I feel exposed. Confidence falls from me. I fiddle nervously with the crop still under my clothing. They begin. The sound of their strikes fills the room. I study my friend apprehensively, but she has found her state of ecstasy. I'm ready to fade into the crowd.

The eyes of the raven-haired mistress catch me. Invitingly, she holds out her hand. I shake my head instinctively. Her offer remains.

Something within me changes. I feel desire coursing. I pull the crop out from my clothing. I have always considered myself to be a sexually confident person, but as I stand over my friend, hesitating, I am aware for the first time of my internalized shame and pervading insecurities surrounding kink play. My computer screen had been my security blanket, allowing me to explore the world but never fully accept it. What I realized that night is that these points of vulnerability can be transformed into our greatest sources of sexual empowerment—sometimes it just takes whipping your best friend in front of a crowd before you can see it.

The dominatrices smile and step to the side. I raise the crop and strike. It feels dirty, wrong; I let the feeling consume me. My friend and I burst into laughter. We continue, experiencing the strangest duality of hilarity and erotic pleasure. We leave the venue soon after, unable to wipe the smiles off our faces. We have both faced a fear in ourselves—one we didn't even realize was there—and we have won.

I went back to the same club after the pandemic, again under the guise of research for my writing; something that, as my friend pointed out, was sounding ever more like a convenient excuse. The only thing that really shocked me this time was quite how much she had grown. She had spent the past few years purposefully exploring her sexuality and was a completely different person from the one I had known before. There were no awkward giggles and no flushed faces, and certainly no need for a collar to hide behind. There was just pure confidence, in her presence, in her desires, in her limitations. I had come looking for something new and shocking; I didn't expect to find it in the same familiar person I saw every other week.

Kinky Clothing

L eather is one of the fetishes intimately tied to explorations of homosexuality, power play, and gender roles. It is widely considered one of the more popular fetish interests, with an estimated 14.7 percent of the population enjoying the erotic properties of cow's skin. This a fantastic example of how fetishes can be influenced by cultural factors—such as a world war.

The rise of motorcycle gangs across America in the 1940s and '50s has generally been recognized as connected with the return of war veterans. This community and its activities aided veterans in their return from the war: the adrenaline-fueled riding, heavy drinking, and access to the homosocial network that had been established in their years at war were ways they could ease the unreality of "normal" home life after the trauma of combat. Leather was the uniform of biker gangs for practical reasons: the armor-like protection it offered in the event of a fall. Leather had also been a vital part of soldiers' uniforms during the war, when it could be obtained, providing both warmth and, again, protection.

This hypermasculine aesthetic was popularized in Hollywood, and adopted by heartthrob actors of the time such as Marlon Brando and James Dean. This likely cemented leather's association with both masculinity and queer culture, as both Dean and Brando were figures who acknowledged their homosexual desires and behaviors; as Brando famously remarked in an interview in 1976, "Homosexuality is so much in fashion, it no longer makes news. Like a large number of men, I, too, have had homosexual experiences, and I am not ashamed."

Ultimately, leather fashion became a symbol of resistance. It resonated with returned veterans who struggled to reintegrate, and equally with emerging queer subcultures who were tired of hiding their identities from the world. It's likely that its connection with military uniforms and personnel influenced its association with the kink scene, the association with discipline and hierarchy slipping into the homosexual subculture of dominance and submission. The artwork of Tom of Finland truly emphasizes this fact, as his homoerotic drawings often depict men partly clothed in leather caps, jackets, or pants.

By the end of the 1950s, gay leather bars and gay motorcycle clubs began to appear around America. By 1964, *Life* would release an article titled "Homosexuality in America," with pictures of leather-clad gay men in these bars showing the public that queer culture could also be linked to a hypermasculine aesthetic. Over time, this subculture became less associated with its biker foundations and more inclusive of the wider queer community, with activists proposing the inclusion of women by the 1970s. We do, however, continue to pay homage to these origins (and efforts for wider inclusion) today. Each year, Sydney's internationally famous Gay and Lesbian Mardi Gras is opened by Dykes on Bikes, an Australian motorcycle group for queer women that originated in America during this time.

Leather is not the only popular fetish item influenced by World War II. Many believe it was also responsible for a clothing that attracts even more interest—nylon. In 1939, the first pair of women's stockings made from this synthetic material was presented at the New York World's Fair. It would be received with such popularity that the product would simply be known as "nylons." The immense interest that nylon or stocking fetishes have received subverts the assumption that these sexual desires must be rooted in our biology. Less than a hundred years after its release, nylon would become one of the most popular fetishes in the Western world: the fourth most prevalent fetish in Belgium's population, for example—behind more obvious interests, such as lingerie (71.7 percent), breasts (65.5 percent), and buttocks (64.5 percent)—with 29.5 percent claiming to have a particular sexual interest in nylon. Akin to lingerie, the stocking would gain a cultural association with sexuality due to the fact it was technically an undergarment. With fashion of the time generally finishing the skirt below the knee, being able to see the garter would generally happen only during something a little more frisky.

However, there has to be more going on. Stockings existed before this, generally made of silk, but they never experienced the same height of fetishization. As Susannah Handley writes in her book, *Nylon: The Story of a Fashion Revolution* (1999):

> *Nylon became a household word in less than a year and, in all the history of textiles, no other product has enjoyed the immediate, overwhelming public acceptance of DuPont nylon.*

Military parachutes, too, were initially made from silk, a material that had to be imported. As the success of its stockings had demonstrated, DuPont had created a synthetic alternative that could be made on American shores. But soon all its nylon production was reallocated to the war effort, creating the materials for parachutes, tires, and even ammunition bags. New and used stockings were donated to help with the effort. Where 90 percent of DuPont's nylon had been going toward stockings, 100 percent of it was now going toward war material.

As human history will constantly attest, the more we are told we can't have something, the more we want it.

A black market for nylons appeared. Previously sold for $1.15 a pair, they shot up to $20. According to the Chemical Heritage Foundation (now the Science History Institute), one person alone made over $100,000 in sales of diverted nylons. Some of the women who couldn't get their hands on a pair resorted to painting their legs, even drawing seams down the back. Nylon stockings became one of the prime targets for theft. One case of robbery was actually dismissed as a possible motive in a murder investigation due to the fact that no nylon stockings had been taken from the house. This shortage was also being felt in the UK. As American troops were the only people who had (legal) access to nylons, and demand for the product was bordering on desperate, stockings made for the perfect gift if you wanted to woo your British girlfriend while positioned overseas. It's fair to say that, by this stage, nylon stockings had become a fetishized object of nearly everyone's desire.

The drama would only increase when nylons returned to the market in 1945. Cue the "nylon riots." After the war, the stockings were marketed as a symbol of peace, with DuPont announcing the return to production with the slogan "Peace, It's Here! Nylons on Sale!" However, every time stocks of nylons appeared, so did crowds of thousands upon thousands of women. One of the most disruptive riots broke out in Pittsburgh, after forty thousand women had lined up to purchase one of the thirteen thousand pairs available. Riots and disruptions continued until production levels were able to return to prewar quantities. Finally, everyone was able to get their nylons before Christmas.

I doubt that many of us today attach such connotations to stockings, an accessory now thought of as lingerie rather than an everyday essential, but its continued dominance of the erotic landscape goes to show how cultural associations can be passed on through generations. When we see nylons today, we may shout many things, but I doubt that "Peace, it's here!" is one of them.

What I find particularly interesting about the nylon fetish is that despite its prevalence, it is unknown compared with leather or foot fetishes. Now, this is not to say that the more widely known foot fetish does not enjoy far-reaching popularity, though studies into the prevalence of kinks and fetishes generally place nylon higher. I would imagine, however, that these two fetishes may be related.

Nylon, being a relatively recent phenomenon, may be connected to a sexual interest that is far more established—which is not to say, however, that it has been normalized. The virtual world has provided a new avenue for those who have a special interest in feet to explore this desire. Back in 2015, one anonymous foot-fetishist expressed this sentiment in an interview with *Vice*: "The fetish for me is more online than in real life. Mainly because in real life you may run into issues (i.e., a woman may not share your fetish). I'm very private about it, because most people simply don't feel the same way." If, by some miracle of fate, this book manages to make its way into the hands (or feet) of this anonymous fetishist, I would like to assure them that the erotic desire is anything but uncommon.

Foot Fetishes

The Toe-Between

F oot fetishism may well be one of the most enduring fetishes across all of human history. According to data collected by Dr. Justin Lehmiller, one in seven people today have had a sexual fantasy in which feet or toes played a prominent role.[*] The fantasy was most common among gay and bisexual men (21 percent), followed by heterosexual men (18 percent), lesbian and bisexual women (15 percent), and finally heterosexual women (5 percent). The ongoing prevalence of foot fetishes can be demonstrated by the viral appearance of the "vajankle" back in 2015. In case you missed the headlines, the vajankle is a sex toy that is pretty much what you may expect from the name—a vagina in an ankle. This product was designed by Sinthetics back in 2013, after one customer repeatedly contacted the company to ask for it. A handmade silicone foot, with a silicone vagina where the ankle should be, was placed on the market, complete with customizable skin tones and nail polish colors.

That seventh person in every friend group (check their bedside drawer for a vajankle) is far from alone in fantasizing about little piggies going off to market—the fascination is one of the oldest recorded fetishes in history. As stated by Dr. William A. Rossi, a man who spent his life dedicated to shoe design and manufacturing:

---

[*] Lehmiller also states, "It's important to note that just because someone has fantasized about feet before doesn't necessarily mean that they have a fetish for feet. . . . So while about 1 in 7 people reported having had a foot fantasy before, the number who have a true fetish for feet, in the sense of being primarily or only attracted to feet, is likely much smaller than that." Zachary Zane and Justin Lehmiller, "How Common Are Foot Fetishes, and Why Do People Have Them?," *Men's Health*, October 7, 2020, https://menshealth.com/sex-women/a19523651/foot-fetish/.

The foot is an erotic organ and the shoe is its sexual covering. This is a reality as ancient as [hu]mankind, as contemporary as the Space Age. The human foot possesses a natural sexuality whose powers have borne remarkable influence on all peoples of all cultures throughout all history.

There was a clear recognition of the erotic properties of feet in ancient Greece. In Hesiod's story of the birth of Aphrodite, the goddess of sexual love and beauty, only one physical attribute is described—her shapely feet, under which grass springs to life as she walks. Descriptions of beautiful, slender, or fine ankles appeared in literature across ancient Greece: Danaë's in the *Iliad*, Ino's in the *Odyssey*, and Alcmene's in the Hesiodic *Scutum*. If there was any existing doubt of the prevalence of foot fetishes, the love letters attributed to the philosopher Philostratus certainly put them all to rest. In his letter "To a Barefoot Boy," Philostratus worships the shape of his lover's feet and implores them to always walk barefoot so that he may kiss the footprints left behind:

O' perfect lines of feet most dearly loved!
O' flowers new and strange! O' plants sprung from earth!
O' kiss left lying on the ground!

Similar pleas are also made in his letter "To a Woman," whose recipient is similarly urged to keep her feet always bare for the lovers who may want to kiss and worship them:

Do not torture your feet, my love, and do not hide them . . .
walk softly and leave prints of your own foot behind you,
for those who would love to kiss them.

Things take a slightly kinkier turn once we get to his thirty-seventh letter, in that Philostratus describes the feet of a woman that are even better than those of Aphrodite (removing any doubt that the goddess's feet were sexualized at the time) and wishes he could be dominated by these feet.

O' thrice charmed would I be and blessed,
if you [feet] would tread on me.

Way beyond the bedroom, worship of feet has played a prominent role in public life. The emergence of foot washing as a custom is a prime example. Have you heard the story of Jesus washing the feet of his disciples?

> *If I then, your Lord and Teacher, have washed your feet, you also ought to wash one another's feet. For I have given you an example, that you should do as I have done to you.*

In many civilizations, foot washing was a gesture of humility, intimately tied to displays of reverence and love, and generally reserved for the "lower"-standing party to perform upon the person of more authority. During his reign in the ninth century, Pope Eugene II asked his adherents to kiss his feet, a custom that continues to be practiced today.

In the century following, foot binding began in China under Emperor Li Yu. He is said to have been entranced by a court dancer, Yao Niang, who bound her feet into the shape of a moon and danced on her toes inside a six-foot golden lotus. This obsession was sexual from the beginning and was quickly taken up by ladies of the court as a symbol of high-status feminine refinement. Indeed, it had a profound impact on the course of women's lives and their "marriageability." The coveted foot size, the "golden lotus," was three inches. For context, most iPhones today are closer to five. Four-inch feet, "silver lotuses," were acceptable. However, women who could not get their feet smaller than five inches were dismissed as "iron lotuses" and their marriage prospects fell to next to none.

And this is not ancient history. The last shoe factory making lotus shoes only ceased production in 1999.

With one in seven individuals under the erotic spell of feet, it is safe to bet that many well-known historical figures were inflicted with this passion. Shall we go and see for ourselves?

The man in question must still be hiding away with Joyce (hopefully not collaborating on any fart-focused letters). Let us try to find him!

F. Scott Fitzgerald, the author of *The Great Gatsby* (1925), was likely one such devotee. Fitzgerald repeatedly visited one sex worker because of her feet, and was even described by her as a "foot fetishist." While he loved feet (or at least the feet of this particular woman), he detested his own and refused to let anyone see them naked. He admitted that he was plagued by a "Freudian shame about his feet."

Our good friend Freud had two insightful takes on foot fetishes. As with all things Freud, it had to do with either the penis or wanting to fuck your mom. This is one of the fortunate times when we find ourselves in the middle of this Venn diagram. One theory proposed that lusting after feet was common because it was the most likely part of your mom's body to see naked—a child might sneak into her bedroom and see a foot poking out from the covers, and thus form erotic connotations. His second theory was simpler: that feet and toes resemble the shape of the penis. (I honestly believe it would be hard to find a part of the body that Freud does *not* think looks like the penis.)

More recently, a researcher, completely by accident, stumbled upon another theory. In 1999, neuroscientist Vilayanur Subramanian Ramachandran was studying phantom limb syndrome, a condition in which amputees can still feel, and believe they can move, their missing limbs. He determined that the syndrome resulted from the fact that the brain, which contains effectively a map of the body, sometimes fails to erase body parts that have been removed. Here's where things get a little more complicated: for some of the phantom-foot patients, the brain didn't just fail to erase the missing foot from its map—it rewired the map in a way that caused sexual stimulation. Now, the area of the somatosensory cortex responsible for feeling in the feet is very close to the one responsible for genitalia. Ramachandran thus felt confident in proposing that the reason for this sexual fetish could be because those sections of the brain commonly become "cross-wired." He stated, "Maybe even many of us so-called normal people have a bit of cross-wiring, which would explain why we like to have our toes sucked." While this theory is yet to be proven as fact (and has been the subject of much debate), it does provide an interesting example of how fetishes and sexual desires may have a biological underpinning. The practice of reflexology offers another example of how the body can be aroused, sexually or otherwise, by stimulating the feet—with certain spots on the foot believed to correlate to genital areas when massaged (a phenomenon now colloquially referred to as a "footgasm").

There are external factors that may have impacted the foot fetish, too. One compelling study from 1998 found a connection with four major sexually transmitted epidemics in history: gonorrhea in the thirteenth century, syphilis in the sixteenth and nineteenth centuries, and AIDS in the late twentieth century. Researchers determined that during each of those periods, a sexual focus on the female foot emerged in literature, the press, and other media. In the thirteenth century, it showed up in romantic literature and troubadour poetry. In the sixteenth century, a movement in popular fashion drew eroticized attention to women's feet; the term *toe-cleavage* became used to describe shoes that displayed the base of the first two toes. By the nineteenth century, brothels began to specialize in foot eroticization on a large scale. It wasn't until the 1980s, however, that the connection between foot fetishes and the contemporary epidemic was explicitly recognized. As foot pornography emerged in magazines, some editorials advertised that "foot-sex" could be regarded as a pleasurable, safe alternative to penetrative sex, which ran the risk of STIs.

After completing their review of historical literature, the researchers of this study went on to review issues from eight of the largest pornographic magazines in the United States, released between 1965 and 1994. Their investigation revealed that the number of foot-oriented pictures had *soared* over the course of the AIDS epidemic. At the time of their study, in 1998, it showed no sign of slowing down; however, they predicted that "this general interest in foot-fetishism will decline when the AIDS epidemic subsides," following the same pattern they had discerned from previous pandemics. With this period of history not long behind us, it's not really a wonder that when Justin Lehmiller discovered his one-in-seven statistic, he found that the highest demographic of people who had fantasied about feet was queer men (21 percent).

Now, in themselves, these facts are fascinating—but when put together, they tell a bigger story. That a sexual desire that is shared so widely could have a biological or cultural basis should be the subject of fascination and intellectual interest. With that said, the attempts over the years to formulate theories about the origins of many kinks and fetishes should be treated with caution. This impulse to find definitive causes for our desires is part of a broader trend in sexual research, and one that shouldn't be entered into lightly—while the search for causes or origins can be presented as a desire to better understand kinks and fetishes, it can also come from a desire to eradicate them. A similar double-edged-sword scenario presented itself in the search for the "gay gene," which began in the latter half of the twentieth century. For some, this was perceived as an effort to legitimize queer sexualities, demonstrating that homosexuality was part of one's DNA. Others saw the insidious potential for such research to be misused, fearing an underlying eugenicist impulse toward eradicating homosexuality—because if we are able to isolate the cause, we are able to "fix" the problem.

Understandably, a cause-and-effect theory can appear more attractive at first glance, appeasing our need for neat, logical answers. When it comes to fetishes, however, I think we need to come to a more fluid version of sexuality—one that not only tolerates, but embraces the various "kinks" in our vision of desire. A range of aspects may come into play—biological, cultural, environmental, and psychological.

Indeed, how much more could we learn about the function of a human if we stopped treating these desires as "freaky quirks" and instead worked to show that they function in a holistic view of a human? What if, as with eating and sleeping, we recognized that there are nature/nurture factors that influence our preferences, our likes and dislikes? If someone said they preferred eating in a quiet pub to dining in an overcrowded bar, or sleeping with one pillow rather than one under every limb, we would not bat an eyelid. Yet when someone tells us it takes having their toes sucked to get them in the mood, it's likely to end up on some Reddit forum. Why is it that our kinky inclinations have come to be clouded in so much shame?

Crime and Pleasurable Punishment

B y this time in the evening, you will be entirely unsurprised to learn that our thinking about sex changed significantly as we came into the nineteenth century. Prior to this, we had no word to conceptualize a sexual practice that deviated from what was "normal," even though these behaviors had always existed. The adoption of an increasingly medicalized worldview at this historical tipping point meant labeling everything as normative or nonnormative, *especially* when it came to sexual behavior.

Look who came running in at our previous mention of Freud! It seems the two stopped bickering long enough for Richard von Krafft-Ebing to prick up his ears.

Krafft-Ebing was incredibly influential in this field. His 1886 publication, *Psychopathia Sexualis* (*Sexual Psychopathy: A Clinical-Forensic Study*), changed the game when it came to thinking about sexuality. The publication went through twelve editions throughout Krafft-Ebing's lifetime, the final one featuring 238 case histories of sexual behavior. This work is remembered now for giving names to concepts that previously had none, such as homosexuality, bisexuality, sadism, masochism, necrophilia, and anilingus. The uncategorizable had finally been categorized, and Krafft-Ebing's ruling was undoubtedly clear: any sexual act that did not have the intention of procreation was to be considered a perversion (I can hear Aquinas and Augustine murmuring their agreement at the other end of the living room).

With opportunity for the natural satisfaction of the sexual instinct, every expression of it that does not correspond with the purpose of nature—i.e., propagation—must be regarded as perverse.

Yes, this even includes your recreational late-night hookups. Pervert.

So: penetrative, heterosexual, procreative activity was *normal*—and everything else fell into the category of *deviant*. Krafft-Ebing devised the term *sadism* in reference to the infamous French author the Marquis de Sade, whose pornographic works were filled with confronting accounts of sexual violence and torture. *Masochism* was named after Austrian author Leopold von Sacher-Masoch, whose work *Venus in Furs* (1870) shocked readers with its inclusion of a dominatrix-style relationship with a beautiful woman. We will be sure to make the closer acquaintance of these men shortly.

By 1913, the compound usage of the term *sado-masochism* appeared in academic work, as psychoanalysts such as Sigmund Freud and Isidor Isaak Sadger analyzed how these two conditions could be related. But herein lies the problem. When these men decided to put names on these experiences, it wasn't done just in an effort to understand them—it was to diagnose, a step on the path to finding a cure. They defined "normal" by scraping away all the edges and setting aside these offcuts in shame.

Yet, what this neat categorization of normative versus nonnormative fails to capture is that sadomasochistic practices have had their place throughout history. In the ancient world especially, they are almost more prevalent than any conventionally amorous depictions of sex. Inside the remaining Villa of the Mysteries from ancient Pompeii, we can see a winged woman whipping a naked woman engaged in an erotic dance. In the aptly named Tomb of the Whipping from the Etruscan civilization, we can see a depiction of two men spanking and flogging a woman as they mutually pleasure each other. Indic texts such as the *Kama Sutra* (ca. 400 BCE) and the *Koka Shastra* (1150 CE) discuss the use of painful activities—such as spanking, hair pulling, biting, and scratching—to enhance sexual activities.

Erotic strangulation was another fashion that spread through Europe in the eighteenth century. While the practice of flagellation brought with it a range of risks, the rise of strangulation brought much worse. Indeed, accidental deaths due to strangulation in pleasure houses became frequent enough for the courts to attempt to suppress this sexual trend—censoring the details so the general public would not get any ideas. Erotic strangulation also found a home within quasi-medical literature. Just like flagellation, it was advertised as a perfect way to make your little soldier rise and increase fertility.

Check out this pamphlet titled "An Essay on the Art of Strangulation": "Every thing which produced irritation in the lungs and thorax, produced also titulation in the generate organs . . . which animate and invigorate the machinery of procreation." The only way to acquire this wonderful sensation, however, was to hang a man temporarily by rope—an act that landed many of them (such as Peter Motteux and Franz Kotzwara) in early graves, and had many sex workers (such as Susannah Hill) on trial for murder. But this tragic outcome was not enough to stop the erotic trend. As one article from *The Bon Ton Magazine* notes, "The strangulation of Kotzwara, however whimsically fated, has not entirely discouraged the practice"—the reason being that in the "moments before his final exit" he had, in fact, displayed "*certain signs* of ability" that indicated that strangulation was a productive way to get your penis hard (if only he had been cut down in time to use it).

Interest in sadomasochistic practices has shown no sign of petering out. Depictions of consensual violence remain one of the most popular categories of pornography, with 35 percent of people aged fifteen to twenty-nine enjoying these videos. The percentage of people who actually engage in these acts is lower. Back in 1990, *The Kinsey Institute New Report on Sex* stated, "5–10 percent of the US population engages in sadomasochism for sexual pleasure on at least an occasional basis, with most incidents being either mild or staged activities involving no real pain or violence."

This makes sense. There are a number of safety factors to take into consideration when incorporating pain in the bedroom. Without proper education or instruction, many people feel deterred from realizing these fantasies. I would say that this is also one of the more stigmatized forms of kink behavior—and understandably. For those not familiar with the kink scene, the apparent disconnect between important social justice work done to reduce violence in the real world and exploring it consensually can be uncomfortable. This comes down to a vital distinction between reality and fantasy. I have often heard debates surrounding sadomasochistic play equating the act to domestic violence, which reveals a deeply ingrained misunderstanding.

There is an intimate connection between the human experiences of pain and pleasure. On the fundamental level of biology, both cause our central nervous system to release endorphins, chemicals that can induce feelings of euphoria. This is perhaps why when women experience an orgasm, thirty areas of the brain are activated, including those that are involved in pain. Even outside the bedroom, we seek out a range of painful activities for the sake of pleasure. What other reason do we have for eating spicy chili or throwing our fate into the hands of those running pop-up festival roller coasters (these are the people *I* think we need to be concerned about)?

A similar sensation is behind the experience of the runner's high. During a marathon or intense exercise, there comes a time (or so I hear) when the body sends signals to the brain to say it's time to chill out (which is exactly right: go back to bed). However, this experience can be temporarily overwritten by a feeling of euphoria, as endorphins are released to block the pain. Adrenaline is also produced as a result of this pain, adding to the excitement of this blissful high. This pleasurable sensation is the experience that keeps runners and exercise lovers coming back for more. In ye olde times, this was likely a survival mechanism to help our ancestors hunt their prey or escape from predators. Now it is just a mechanism to ensure the rest of us feel bad for not also getting up at six a.m. to jog around in spandex.

The point to all of this—besides exposing my envy of people capable of functioning before nine a.m.—is that pleasurable pain is a distinctly human experience. Professor Paul Rozin even coined the term *benign masochism* to describe our enjoyment of negative sensations when we're aware there is no actual threat to our safety. This is a distinction that other members of the animal kingdom are not cognitively able to make. If you put a cat on a roller coaster, I highly doubt they'd be running back for a ticket to drop two hundred meters in the air again. (And if my experience with Crush's Coaster at Disneyland is enough to go on, that would be a highly logical cat. Never. Again.)

It is this crucial distinction that allows people to enjoy the pleasure that comes from eating ghost peppers, watching scary movies, zooming on a ride at two hundred kilometers per hour, and yes, being whipped in the bedroom. The logic of equating sadomasochism with domestic violence is like comparing eating spicy food to self-harm. Without often realizing it, many of us have participated in popular sexual acts that would be considered sadomasochistic, such as spanking, slapping, choking, and hair pulling.

One recent cultural sensation in particular brought sadomasochism as a BDSM practice into public conversation.

The Fifty Shades trilogy was far more than a set of books on a shelf—it was a phenomenon. The series topped bestseller lists worldwide. By 2017, it had sold over 150 million copies. The cinematic adaptation broke box-office records by bringing in over $81 million during its Valentine's weekend release. Prior to the pandemic, Fifty Shades was the last global phenomenon responsible for a boom in sex toys, and perhaps even conversation around sexual practices.

But as sexy and fun as the whole thing was, it came under heavy criticism from both the BDSM and more conservative communities. For once, voices from these two widely varying ideologies seemed to be arguing the same thing—that the depictions of nonnormative sexual practices in this book were dangerous and should not be romanticized. And on this point, I tend to agree. While it is entirely possible to watch and enjoy "problematic" media while keeping in mind that it is, in fact, problematic, there was something a bit more complex going on. The representation of BDSM practices and a nonnormative relationship was so poor that it arguably did more harm than good. Unless you know how these relationships are ethically managed, it is hard (if not impossible) to recognize the series as problematic while enjoying it—and it was meant to be *educating* the masses on these practices.

Now, I don't believe for a second that this was E. L. James's mission when she started writing her Twilight fan fiction. It was a responsibility that was forced upon the series due to its unprecedented success. Yet, it was a responsibility nonetheless; one that, largely, went unaddressed.

The proof is all in the (very sticky) pudding. The year the book was released, emergency room visits in the US due to BDSM or toy-related injuries increased by 50 percent from the previous year. While this could be accounted for by the equal increase in sex-toy sales, it is far more likely* due to the fact that people were re-creating scenarios they had read without a proper understanding of how to do so safely. Christian Grey may have put ben wa balls and spreader bars into our vocabulary, but he sure as hell didn't teach us how to sanitize them correctly.

So, what do we do with *Fifty Shades of Grey*? Do we burn it and bury it? Put it into the Red Room of Pain and give it a good spanking? When something—a book, film, song, or show—becomes a cultural phenomenon, it is not so much about what we can learn from it, but what the frenzy it causes can teach us about a culture. Fifty Shades didn't become a worldwide craze just because it was scandalous and sexy—it tapped into a desire that had lain dormant in millions upon millions of people.

A more recent comparison could be found in the success of Cardi B's "WAP," a song surrounded in controversy and yet blasted from the speakers of happy dancing millions. Neither the book nor the song is simply offering sex. My guess is that the appeal lies in this: an open *conversation* about sex, representations of different practices and presentations of one's sexuality, and an unapologetic declaration that one can be empowered by sex without being objectified.

For those who didn't end up in an emergency room, there was one benefit that fans of Fifty Shades claimed to reap: an improved sex life, especially for women. I'd speculate it wasn't just the incorporation of fluffy handcuffs that did the trick. Fifty Shades plays with the concept of power—with fantasies of domination, control, and submission—in many ways. Power imbalance is a crucial relationship dynamic in many romantic stories that we have enjoyed throughout the ages (it wasn't just Mr. Darcy's wet shirt, you know). This is what draws audiences in, what captivates us with these couples, even if we don't openly admit it. Fifty Shades brought that tension, bubbling away under every romantic story, to the surface—and not only that, it gave that tension a body. We—and by "we" I mean the audience of mostly women—were invited to get lost in this fantasy of financial, physical, and often emotional domination, and the result, for so many, was a liberating euphoria.

---

* By comparison, the pandemic-induced increase in toy and bondage sales did not lead to a significant increase in these forms of injuries.

There is one line from the books that I believe encapsulates the craze completely. When explaining to Anastasia the ideology of being a submissive (in email format, quite infamously), Christian states they are the ones who truly have all the power:

> *What I think you fail to realize is that in Dom/sub relationships, it is the sub who has all the power. That's you. I'll repeat this—you are the one with all the power. Not I. . . . I can't touch you if you say no—that's why we have an agreement—what you will and won't do. If we try things and you don't like them, we can revise the agreement. It's up to you—not me.*

This is actually in line with observations made by the Kinsey Institute, which remarked that "most often it is the receiver (the masochist), not the giver (the sadist), who sets and controls the exact type and extent of the couple's activities." I imagine this is similar to the experience people had when reading Fifty Shades—empowerment in and control of their own sexuality by allowing themselves to be lost in a fantasy of domination and control.

That being the case, it's truly no wonder that the story struck a chord with so many women across the globe. Someone's fantasies often differ significantly from their everyday behaviors. Indeed, people in high-powered jobs are generally the most likely to fantasize about being submissive. As the Kinsey Institute reported, "in many such heterosexual relationships, the so-called traditional sex roles are reversed—with men playing the submissive or masochistic role." For so many busy mothers and working professionals, the fantasy of being whisked away and freed from decisions, control, and the burden of responsibilities (Anastasia doesn't even need to worry about what to *eat*) is just about as sexy as you could possibly get.

Our fantasy lives and our real lives rarely match up—that's what makes the former so enthralling. This escapism offers its own positive effects once we return to the real world: it is not dissimilar to the experience of many during sexual role-play. In an interview, a US-based dominatrix, Mistress Mean Mommy, compared her exploration of different personae during BDSM play to reading James Joyce's *A Portrait of the Artist as a Young Man* (note: not the fart letters):

*I can't understand what it's like to be a 15-year-old Irish boy in an all-boys'
boarding school. But I can read the book and have a sense of what it's like.
So if you wanna go out and buy a school-boy's uniform and wear it and have
somebody be the school-master and I get to play it, now I have a sense of what
it's like, even as me in my body as a woman. I'll never be a 15-year-old boy. I
get to experience what I think a 15-year-old boy would be like. And that might
be freeing in some way. Maybe it will give me a different perspective. Maybe I'll
suddenly understand something I never understood about young boys.*

The experience of sexual role-play has been understood to offer a possible number
of benefits. In particular, practitioners have praised the insights this play has offered
into their own identities, fleshing out concepts such as gender, age, and sexual orientation. Taking on roles that are completely different from their lives—such as a dominatrix becoming a schoolmaster, or a CEO becoming a sexual submissive—allows people
to venture into an unexplored part of who they are. This exploration can be especially
beneficial for those whose social identity is generally felt to be on the outskirts of social
acceptability. Studies have found role-play to be helpful for members of the queer community, allowing them to reconcile and accept aspects of their identity that had been
laden in cultural shame.

The act of adopting different roles highlights for many the performative character
of gender and sexual identities, providing an insight into the equally performative nature of these roles in the real world. It speaks to fluidity of identity, and the benefit of
viewing it as a mutable and ever-developing part of one's being. Such revelations can
be even more profound than those moments of epiphany gained through reading a
good book. Sexual role-play is, by its nature, an *embodied* experience. The insights and
lessons we gain through this form of experimentation are not only intellectual, but a
felt experience.

Despite the considerable benefits this form of sexual play offers, the number of
people who participate in role-play is considerably lower than those who participate
in acts of BDSM. Only 26 percent of all our survey participants claimed to have role-
played in the previous year. Once again, the number of those who had participated

was noticeably higher for those who were gender diverse; the highest demographic was trans women (42 percent), followed by trans men (33.8 percent) and nonbinary people (31.4 percent). It is perhaps because role-play engages so intimately with ideas of gender performativity and subversion of stereotypes that it appeals strongly to those who must often confront these ideas in their everyday life. Alternatively, it may also be through a heightened participation in role-play that many people have been able to access insights into their own gender identities and expressions.

Role-play is far from a new thing. Long before Christian Grey came on the scene, esteemed authors were already exploring the joys and benefits of being spanked and dominated—perhaps none quite so succinctly as Jean-Jacques Rousseau (1712–1778).

There he is now in the billiards room, concentrating on the game at hand. Rousseau has always been a true lover of games. He believes there is a certain art to them, though one he can never quite put his finger on. Shall we watch now to see who comes out on top?

Rousseau was a Genevan philosopher and writer whose ideas heavily influenced the European enlightenment. While Rousseau would spend years developing his political and economic ideas, his sexual "enlightenment" took place early on. As a young boy, Rousseau found himself under the care of Mademoiselle Lambercier—and, as she "had a mother's affection for us, she also exercised a mother's authority, and sometimes even carried it so far as to chastise us, when we deserved it." It was from his first experience of being punished at the hands of Mademoiselle Lambercier that Rousseau believed he was set for a lifetime of perversity: "Who would believe that this child-punishment, received at eight years old from the hand of a woman of thirty, determined my taste, my desires, my passions, my whole being for the remainder of my life, and that in a manner quite opposite of what might naturally be expected." Even at this young age, Rousseau recognized that his experience of being spanked was perhaps as pleasurable as it was painful. From this first act of discipline, he found himself desirous of again inciting Mademoiselle Lambercier's rage:

> *It required even the whole depth of this affection, added by all my natural gentleness, to prevent me from courting, by fresh offenses, a return of the same treatment; for I had experienced in the smart, in the very shame, a degree*

of sensuality which induced greater desire than fear of experiencing a new infliction from the same hand. 'Tis true that a similar chastisement from her brother would by no means have appeared agreeable, for a certain precocious sexual instinct doubtless entered into the matter.

Rousseau's awareness of his kink at an early age is not dissimilar to the experience of many today; the majority of people (61.4 percent) claim to have become aware of their specific kink or fetish before their twenty-fifth birthdays. To Rousseau's disappointment, however, Mademoiselle Lambercier ceased to administer this punishment once she realized it was not having the desired effect. This would not prevent him from craving this discipline as he matured. Though he tried to fight his sexual desire for spanking, Rousseau could not help it creeping into his romantic imagination.

Long tormented I knew not by what, my eyes gloated on every handsome woman; incessantly did my fancy recall them, simply to turn them to account after my fashion, and transform them into so many Miss Lamberciers.

Rousseau would finally find someone capable of fulfilling his fantasy. Françoise-Louise de Warens (1699–1762)—twelve years Rousseau's senior—lived a liberal lifestyle for a woman of her time. She had first made Rousseau's acquaintance when he was sixteen, converting him to Protestantism during her employment as a political spy (?!), a role she took on after her silk stocking business failed. At the age of twenty, Rousseau returned to her and proposed an affair. As Warens already had another lover, a ménage à trois took shape. She became the great love of Rousseau's life and engaged willingly in his fantasies of power and punishment—she called him "little one" and he called her "Maman." The intoxication of this fantasy was enough for Rousseau to accept (for a while) the discomfort he felt about their three-way relationship.

To fall at the feet of an imperious mistress, to obey her mandates, to be obliged to implore her pardon were to me most exquisite enjoyments, and yet the more my lively fancy inflamed my blood, the more like a bashful lover did I become.

Spanking and domination by a mother figure weren't the only interesting desires Rousseau enjoyed—he also experimented with exhibitionism. It could be said, however, that his desire to expose himself still revolved around his primary fantasy of being spanked by an "imperious mistress." See, Rousseau desired to surprise beautiful ladies with his ass:

> *I sought out dark alleys and secret by-places wherein to expose myself from afar to persons of the other sex in the state I should have liked to be in with them. What they saw was not the obscene object—I did not even think of such a thing—'twas the ridiculous one. The sottish pleasure I took in displaying it to their view is beyond the possibility of description.*

While affording pleasure in itself, this act of exhibitionism was performed in hopes that the woman might be "bold enough" to afford him the treatment he desired most of all—being spanked in that dark alley. You may well ask why a man who was, and is, such a prominent and influential figure would record all these misdemeanors. In fact, Rousseau not only wrote down all of his promiscuous actions and desires, but went so far as to have them published. Toward the end of his life, he wrote an autobiographical work, *Confessions*, which would be published in 1782, after his death. It was his wish to provide an authentic and introspective portrait of who he truly was as a person, and not just as a public figure. As he says:

> *Such are the faults and failings of my youth. I have given their history with a fidelity that pleases my heart. If, in the sequel, I honor my riper years with certain virtues, I shall tell them, too, with the same frankness. And, indeed, such was my design. . . . If the memory of me reach posterity, the world may, perchance, one day learn what I had to say.*

Such an account is certainly fascinating now, providing us an uninhibited insight into the sexual fantasies and desires of one of history's great figures.

But Rousseau was not the only person in this room who enjoyed a bit of S&M play with a beautiful woman. Shall we head over to that table there? To the man sitting next to J. R. R. Tolkien, offering him advice on the map he is creating of Middle Earth. Tolkien's good friend has quite of a lot of experience with fantasy worlds.

Before he became one of the most prolific Christian thinkers of the twentieth century, C. S. Lewis (1898–1963), author of the Chronicles of Narnia, was channeling his inner Anastasia Steele. During his late teens, Lewis reportedly became fascinated with sadomasochistic practices. He read the infamous pornographic works of the Marquis de Sade (him again!), and developed, as one biographer termed it, "mildly sadomasochistic fantasies." In 1917, he wrote letters to his friend Arthur Greeves about these fantasies.

> *Across my knee, of course, makes one think of positions for Whipping: or rather not for whipping (you couldn't get any swing) but for that torture with brushes. This position, with its childish nursery associations, has something beautifully intimate and also very humiliating for the victim.*

He signed these letters as Philomastix, which translates in Greek to "lover of the whip." Akin to Rousseau's, Lewis's fantasies of pain were intimately tied with fantasies of domination—in particular, being dominated by an older, more powerful woman.

Indeed, Lewis would have an ongoing affair with the mother of one of the friends he made during his time serving in World War I. Paddy Moore had asked Lewis to take care of his mother if he did not make it home. Lewis would fulfill this request to its extremes. As it turned out, Paddy Moore's mom did, in fact, have it going on. Lewis moved in with Mrs. Moore after he returned (their relationship beginning before she became divorced). Lewis was nineteen when they first met and Mrs. Moore over forty. Though the suspected affair remains unconfirmed, most signs seem to point to the affirmative—especially in consideration of the kind of letters and fantasies that "Philomastix" over here was writing and entertaining. If Rousseau and Lewis are to be believed, then there is nothing that can bend the will of man more than a beautiful woman capable of inflicting pain.

The Lion, the Witch, and the Dominatrix

The figure of the dominatrix has a long history, arguably dating all the way back to the rituals of the goddess Inanna (or Ishtar) in ancient Mesopotamia. Inanna was associated with love, beauty, sex, and war, and is believed to have been worshipped as early as 4000–3100 BCE. These rituals went a little bit further than just a singsong chant and dance. Hymns to this goddess in ancient texts describe her as a despotic force, capable of forcing both men and gods into submission.

Like a fearsome lion you pacify the insubordinate and unsubmissive with your gall.

To complement this verbal description, Inanna is depicted on a seal from the Akkadian Empire in a pose notably similar to contemporary imaginings of a dominatrix— she stands powerfully in battle gear, wings outstretched, an exposed leg extended so she can tread upon a lion, which she holds tame on a leash. In her book, *The History & Arts of the Dominatrix* (2013), historian Anne O. Nomis writes that rituals of the cult members who worshipped Inanna included cross-dressing and were "imbued with pain and ecstasy, bringing about initiation and journeys of altered states of consciousness; punishment, moaning, ecstasy, lament and song, participants exhausting them-

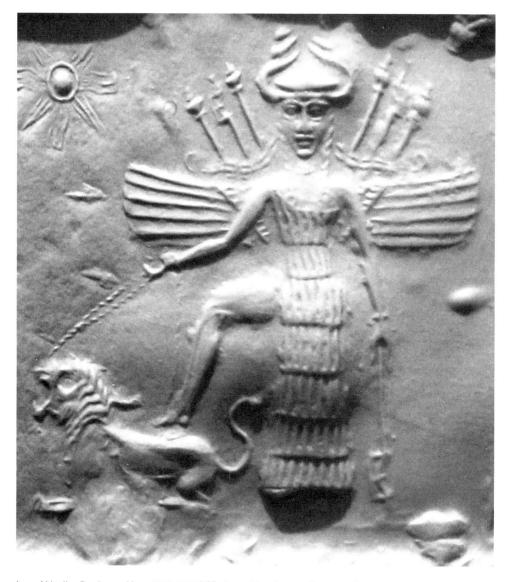

In an Akkadian Empire seal from 2350–2150 BCE, the goddess Inanna showcases her power.

selves with weeping and grief." Inanna became known as the queen of the heavens, choosing whether to inflict pleasure or pain on her subjects.

The dominatrix was born in literature of the tenth century. The canoness Hrotsvitha (935–1001) was the first writer to use the Latin word in her legend "Maria." She claims in the preface that she intended to show the archetypal fragile woman as victorious and the strong man as rooted in confusion—Maria is an "unattainable woman" who rejects all her male suitors. Hrotsvitha was followed by an abundance of literature on courtly love: "a love at once illicit and morally elevating, passionate and disciplined, humiliating and exalting, human and transcendent."

Courtly love was removed from the confines of marriage—which in the medieval period often had very little to do with mutual love and attraction—and consisted of a series of stylized rituals. It took place most often in literature between a knight and a married lady of high rank—beginning a trend of worshipping (read: simping over) an *unattainable lady.* Rather than being seen as an actual living, breathing human, these women were a symbol for everything the knight desired but could not have. While no one was being whipped in latex, courtly love centered on the fantasy of being dominated, spiritually and emotionally, by a beautiful woman. The more obstacles placed in the way, the more he would drool.

Fantasies of cruel love and domination crept through European literature into the early modern period, becoming increasingly explicit. By the seventeenth century, Robert Herrick (1591–1674) was writing poems that wouldn't feel too distant from the likes of *Fifty Shades of Grey* today.

> *Me thought (last night) love in an anger came,*
> *And brought a rod, so whipt me with the same:*
> *Mirtle the twigs were, meerly to imply;*
> *Love strikes, but 'tis with gentle crueltie.*
> *Patient I was: Love pitifull grew then,*
> *And stroak'd the stripes, and I was whole agen.*

Any discussion here needs to include the queen of all dominatrices. Do follow me upstairs to the parlor, toward the sounds of whipping and wailing. You really must meet Theresa Berkley (unknown–1836).

When it comes to BDSM, Mistress Berkley changed the game. In a time when most women were entitled to little, Berkley amassed a fortune running a high-class brothel in the West End of London. This wasn't just any old brothel (if there is such a thing)—Berkley's establishment specialized in flagellation and chastisement. As one source from the time described it:

> Her instruments of torture were more numerous than those of any other governess. Her supply of birch was extensive, and kept in water, so that it was always green and pliant: she had shafts with a dozen whip thongs on each of them; a dozen different sizes of cat-o'-nine-tails, some with needle points worked into them; various kinds of thin bending canes; leather straps like coach traces; battledoors, made of thick sole-leather, with inch nails run through to docket, and currycomb tough hides rendered callous by many years flagellation. Holly brushes, furze brushes; a prickly evergreen, called butcher's brush; and during the summer, glass and China vases, filled with a constant supply of green nettles, with which she often restored the dead to life. Thus, at her shop, whoever went with plenty of money, could be birched, whipped, fustigated, scourged, needle-pricked, half-hung, holly-brushed, furze-brushed, butcher-brushed, stinging-nettled, curry-combed, phlebotomized, and tortured till he had a belly full. . . . Mrs. Berkley had also in her second floor, a hook and pulley attached to the ceiling, by which she could draw a man up by his hands. This operation is also represented in her memoirs.

Far more than just a collector, Berkley was an inventor of kinky devices. In fact, she invented one device that is almost certain to be found in any kink dungeon today: the Berkley Horse, a triangular frame to which a person can be tied, leaving their backside exposed. Henry Spencer Ashbee describes it thus:

> It is capable of being opened to a considerable extent, so as to bring the body to any angle that might be desirable. There is a print in Mrs. Berkley's memoirs, representing a man upon it quite naked. A woman is sitting in a chair exactly under it, with her bosom, belly, and bush exposed: she is manualizing his embolon, whilst Mrs. Berkley is birching his posteriors.

Her establishment became known as the Horse for this reason. The device became so infamous that the Royal Society of Arts even took possession of the original after her death. Though Berkley was renowned for her unparalleled flogging abilities, she would, if the price was right, let customers return the favor.

> *There were, of course, provisions for those who preferred to do the flogging, rather than to receive it. If the price was right, Mrs. Berkeley herself would submit, but if the customer was a glutton, she had several women in her employ who would take anything the client wished to offer short of death. Some of these young ladies bore such colorful nicknames as One-Eyed Peg and Ebony Bet.*

Many a prominent figure was tied to the horse in the Horse. Most notably, King George IV was a frequent patron, who is believed to have enjoyed having his ass tortured by Berkley herself. With benefactors like this, besides the obvious financial advantage, Berkley kept herself safe from the law—and it would have helped that many prominent lawmakers and enforcers took their turns tied to her horse.

Theresa Berkley became such a notorious and intriguing figure in London that she was even impersonated in a publication. *Exhibition of Female Flagellants in the Modest and Incontinent World* (1830) was an anonymously published pornographic novel that many attributed to Berkley, the reigning queen of the female flagellant world. On the cover, the novel claims to "[Prove] from Indubitable Facts, That a Number of Ladies Take a Secret Pleasure, in Whipping Their Own, and Children Committed to Their Care." To build this case, the author includes a series of segments from letters that they claim to have come "from Authentic Anecdotes, French and English, Found in a Lady's Cabinet." These letters expose a range of stories and interactions in which women from all walks of life partake in this fashionable vice—schoolteachers and mothers, workers and royalty. Even nuns are guilty.

> *On the continent, where whipping is so fashionable, it is one of the chief amusements of the Nuns, for they not only whip one another for their pleasure, but will whip with shocking birch-rods their boarders, with so much severity, that*

sometimes some of them are obliged to keep their beds for two or three days . . .
some Nuns take as much pleasure in whipping . . . as they would almost to
sleep with a man, and have almost the same pleasure.

Flagellation took such a strong hold on the English public during this time that it became known as "the English vice." While spanking was primarily a (destructive) form of corporal punishment in schools and homes, it also seeped heavily into erotic thought. So much so that medical explanations for the connection between flagellation and sexual pleasure were being sought as early as the seventeenth century. One theory was that spanking could be a corrective for male impotence, helping to circulate blood flow and allowing a man to stay hard. Johann Heinrich Meibom (1590–1655), a German doctor, wrote about this theory in his essay *On the Use of Rods in Venereal Matters and in the Office of the Loins and Reins.*

I further conclude that Strokes upon the Back and Loins, as Parts appropriated
for the Generating of the Seed, and carrying it to the Genitals, warm and in-
flame those Parts, and contribute very much to the irritation of Lechery. From
all which, it is no wonder that such shameless wretches, Victims of a detested
appetite, such as we have mention'd, or others by too frequent a Repetition, the
Loins and their vessels being drains have sought for a remedy by FLOGGING.

Thus spanking became so much more than a sometimes pleasurable punishment—it became a quasi-medical treatment. A strong connection between "medical" texts and pornography emerged, a topic we will discuss in more detail once we have finished with our fun and games here. Cloaking sexually imaginative scenes as a "discussion" of sexual perversions and cures was a fantastic way for many writers to avoid censorship and prosecution; Edmund Curll defended himself for publishing the essay above by stating, "The Fault is not in the Subject Matter, but the Inclination of the Reader, that makes these Pieces offensive." Translation: If you are turned on by detailed descriptions of men getting spanked by their wives and became erect as a result, that is on you. This scene was simply described for the sake of #science.

Scenes of flagellation crept into all corners of the literary world. By the nineteenth century, the book collector Henry Spencer Ashbee declared:

> *No English bawdy book is free from descriptions of flagellation, and numerous separate plates exist, depicting whipping scenes; it has caused the separation of man and wife; the genteelest female schools have been made subservient to the passions of its votaries; and formally it was spoken without reserve on the public stage.*

One of the most infamous scenes of flagellation came in John Cleland's *Memoirs of a Woman of Pleasure* (1749). Later in the novel, Fanny Hill, a London sex worker, is asked to serve a client "under the tyranny of a cruel taste"—a predilection for whipping. Fanny's client is plagued by an "ardent desire, not only of being unmercifully whipp'd himself, but of whipping others." This desire, previously unknown to Fanny, intrigues her so much that she willingly submits to his requests. She leads her client to a long bench, and the two role-play a scenario in which the client is being tied down against his will: they "play'd at forcing him to lie down which, after some little show of reluctance, for form's sake, he submitted to." Once he's tied down tightly to the bench, Fanny chooses her whipping device and begins to lash her client across his buttocks.

> *Seizing now one of the rods, I stood over him, and, according to his direction, gave him, in one breath, ten lashes with much good-will, and the utmost nerve and vigour of arm that I could put to them, so as to make those fleshy orbs quiver again under them.... I viewed intently the effect of them, which to me at least appeared surprisingly cruel: every lash had skimmed the surface of those white cliffs, which they deeply reddened, and lapping round the side of the furthermost from me, cut, specially, into the dimple of it, such livid weals, as the blood either spun out from, or stood in large drops on; and, from some of the cuts, I picked out even the splinters of the rod that had stuck in the skin.*

Fanny's client would likely classify as one of Dr. Meibom's "Victims of a detested appetite . . . [who] have sought for a remedy by FLOGGING." He is to be pitied, rather than condemned, for his desire to be whipped. It is an unfortunate deformity of taste for which he is not to be blamed: beyond his power of control, he is "enslaved to so peculiar a taste . . . that render'd him incapable of receiving any pleasure till he submitted to these extraordinary means of procuring it at the hands of pain." In this scene, however, Fanny also makes mention of the other class of people who are afflicted with this unfortunate desire—the people Dr. Meibom determined to have brought about this perverted desire by "too frequent a Repetition" of pleasurable activities.

Age was often considered to be relevant here. Indeed, elderly men were generally depicted to submit themselves to flogging as a necessity to get their "little man" working. Ned Ward's *The London Spy*, a monthly periodical beginning in 1704, makes mention of the fact that "the rod" was in high demand for elderly gentlemen who frequented brothels: "sober Citizen[s] . . . about the Age of Sixty" would inquire after "Learned Students in the Science of Debauchery, *Flogging Cullies*." The same logic appears in Fanny's tale, nearly fifty years later. Fanny states that many men, by virtue of their age, are "obliged to have recourse to this experiment, for quickening the circulation of their sluggish juices, and determining a conflux of the spirits of pleasure towards those flagging, shrively parts, that rise to life only by virtue of those titillating ardours created by the discipline of their opposites, with which they have so surprising a consent." The belief that a good spanking could help men stay hard was a persistent and widespread belief throughout the eighteenth century.

There was another scandalous aspect to this scene of Fanny Hill's: while she was whipping (and being whipped by) her client, she was being watched by her madame through a peephole: "as I well knew Mrs. Cole was an eye-witness . . . to the whole of our transaction." Voyeurism, which has been an unflinchingly popular kink across history, describes a sexual thrill of watching someone, either with or without their knowledge, in a state of undress or engaged in sexual activities. The persistence of this desire can be seen in *Gardens of Pleasure*, a collection of erotic Chinese art that was collected by Ferdinand Bertholet. Erotic art emerged in the Han Dynasty

(206 BCE–220 CE) and would become truly widespread by the tenth century in China. Very often, scenes that depicted couples (both homosexual and heterosexual) in the act would also feature "peep-tom" characters looking on from behind curtains and through windows. Especially from the sixteenth to the eighteenth century, a trend in this erotic art emerges of capturing women in a state of undress, who appear to gaze seductively at the viewer. Along with sadism and masochism, voyeurism would be classified as a sexual perversion in the early twentieth century. Despite attempts to treat it, this sexual interest is still going strong—perhaps best known to us today in the figure of the cuckold.

Let us take a peep into our final room.

One Flew over
the Cuckold's Nest

Now a popular category on any pornography site,* the "cuckold" found its origins in the thirteenth century. The word first appears in the English language in 1250 within the anonymous poem "The Owl and the Nightingale."

There's no man who can't lead his wife astray with this kind of behavior; she can be ill-treated so often that she resolves to satisfy her own needs. God knows, she can't help it if she makes him a cuckold . . . there are plenty of men like this, who can't treat a wife properly; no man is allowed to talk to her; he thinks she'll instantly commit adultery if she looks at a man or speaks politely to him. He keeps her under lock and key; adultery often happens as a result.

The term was derived from the cuckoo bird, a creature who has a habit of laying her eggs in the nests of other birds, to describe a man made foolish by his wife's infidelity. By the sixteenth to seventeenth century, it's fair to say that Europe was *obsessed* with cuckolding. Calling a man a *cuck* or *cuckold* was the most popular—and offensive—

* In 2017, Pornhub Insights reported that every month, 1.75 million people searched for cuckold porn and that it had grown in popularity by 57 percent between 2013 and 2016. And it continues to grow: the latest Pornhub annual review noted that searches for "cuck" and "cuckold" grew by 18 percent during 2022.

insult. A gender alternative, *cuckquean*, also came on the market, in 1562 (#equality), though it didn't enjoy the same degree of usage.

At some stage, the figure of the cuckold was also linked with horns—literary and artistic depictions of men who had unwittingly grown horns of shame atop their heads become increasingly common across European countries. There is ambiguity as to how this came about: some suggest they were ram's horns, which indicate the presence of a challenge during "mating season," or that they were the horns of an ox (a castrated bull) to depict their emasculation; others have suggested the connection to the powdered rhinoceros horns that were sold as an aphrodisiac in Asia, or they were perhaps a visual depiction of the devil and sin. Whatever the reason, many of the terms that link infidelity to horns continue to be prevalent in language today: in Portugal, *cabrão* (big goat) is used to insult a man whose wife is unfaithful, and *poner los cuernos* is a Spanish expression that means "to put horns" (to cheat) on someone. Once you become aware of the meaning, you see it *everywhere*.

In Shakespeare's *Much Ado about Nothing*, Beatrice talks about the fact that if God were to send her a husband, he would almost certainly send a pair of horns as well (implying she will make a cuckold out of him).

there will the Devil meet
me, like an old cuckold, with horns on his head

We find the figure in Chaucer's *The Canterbury Tales*:

> *This carpenter hadde wedded newe a wyf,*
> *Which that he lovede moore than his lyf;*
> *Of eighteteene yeer she was of age.*
> *Jalous he was, and heeld hire narwe in cage,*
> *For she was wylde and yong, and he was old*
> *And demed hymself been lik a cokewold.*
> *(This carpenter had recently wedded a wife,*
> *Whom he loved more than his life;*

She was eighteen years of age.
Jealous he was, and held her narrowly in confinement,
For she was wild and young, and he was old
And believed himself likely to be a cuckold.)

While Bottom the ass is not a horned creature, I think we can also see Shakespeare playing with the cuckold legend in *A Midsummer Night's Dream*. To humiliate his "disobedient" wife, Titania, the fairy king Oberon orders she be placed under the thrall of a spell that will cause her to fall in love with the first person she sees—which happens to be a man who has been charmed to possess the head of a donkey (perhaps the fairy version of the human's horned figure). The fairy queen thus becomes infatuated and sleeps with this appropriately named Bottom. Humiliated upon being released from the spell, Titania has learned her lesson and reunites with her ethically appalling husband:

My Oberon! what visions have I seen!
Methought I was enamour'd of an ass.

Who said that doing it in the ass can't save a marriage?

Think back to your own school days (or perhaps just to a recent drunk evening with friends). Everyone is huddled together, your camera-shy friend has offered to take a picture, someone decides on a random (and difficult-to-say-in-unison) word to say on the count of three. Just as you're doing the countdown, the urge strikes you, an urge stronger than any eleven-year-old can resist . . . You make "bunny ears" behind the head of your poor friend, Jeffrey, and spoil what might otherwise have been a lovely group picture.

But while the "bunny ears" photobomb is a playful (if highly annoying) trend today, it was once far from innocent. In fact, if you were caught pulling the bunny ears out on someone in the sixteenth century, you could well find yourself on the dueling ground.

Making the symbol of horns at someone was yet another way to brand them as a cuckold. In François Bunel's (1522–1599) painting *Actors of the Commedia dell'Arte*, we can see the trickster character placing "bunny ears" (cuckold horns) behind the unwitting man next to him, while making a silly face at the painter, much to the amusement of the other figures. The painting can feel jarring to us today—if you place it next to any group photo, there is an uncanny similarity. The largest difference, however, is that when we sneak bunny ears behind Jeffrey, we don't mean to imply his partner is regularly cheating on him and he is a fool for not seeing the truth. This photobomb hasn't lost its original connotations everywhere.

It may also be the case that this connection of horns with sex brought us one modern term that remains in frequent circulation: *horny*. In the late eighteenth century, the phrase "having the horn" became connected to becoming aroused (and thus a man's "horn" appearing), with *horny* as its own word appearing in the eighteenth century. It's more than plausible that "the horn" became used in this context because the likes of Shakespeare were throwing around phrases such as "thou wouldst be horn-mad" in connection with extramarital sex in the centuries before. And I truly hope that from now on you think about, and are grateful to, the esteemed English bard every time you are horny.

While few people have gone on, as far as I know, to actually grow horns from their heads, the figure of the cuckold has helped to inspire some fetish items still worn today, such as the chastity belt. This underwear-style belt is most often marketed to men, and locks up the wearer's penis, preventing them from getting a full erection or using their genitals until the "key holder" allows. These devices are generally part of BDSM play revolving around orgasm control and "cock and ball" torture, a practice that is very much as it sounds. This fantasy of control—of locking up a partner's genitals until permission is given to release them—has fascinated us for centuries.

While today it is associated with men, the historical fantasy revolved around a woman wearing the belt. Consider the medieval chastity belt. It is likely that you have come across these truly terrifying devices before, either in museums or posted in various corners of the internet. These heavy metal devices look more suitable for chopping a limb off than wearing as an undergarment. This iron "underwear" was supposedly fastened and locked around a woman's waist, with only the husband or father possessing the key, to preserve her purity. The belts came in many different designs; some were made of leather rather than metals (a far more comfortable alternative). Some came with spikes and traps to fight off possible suitors. Those with more lavish tastes could commission a chastity belt decorated with hearts and flowers, and even a convenient hole for the husband to slip in, kept safe by lock and key. For anyone who has ever laid eyes on these horrifying relics, one question (out of many) occupies the mind: How the fuck did women pee?

Well, in a rather enjoyable plot twist, it is likely that these "medieval" chastity belts weren't invented until the nineteenth century—and the reason for their invention was anything but pure. Academic Albrecht Classen set the truth of these torturous devices straight in his work *The Medieval Chastity Belt: A Myth-Making Process* (2007). Literary references to chastity belts have been around since the first millennium, functioning primarily as theological metaphors about the protection of women's virginity—certainly nothing to be taken literally. In 1405, we find one of the earliest images of one of these belts in Konrad Kyeser's *Bellifortis*, an illustrated treatise on military technologies.

Does this mean these belts existed around this time? Not quite. See, there were a few other questionable devices in this manual—such as a transportation device run solely on fart power and a recipe for invisibility. Had these devices been invented, we would simultaneously have been able to solve the climate crisis and make Harry Potter's cloak a lot less cool.

In our teaching of history, we tend to forget that our ancestors had a sense of humor as well—and nothing gets the party a-pumping harder than a filthy sex joke. That is, most likely, all chastity belts were—a humorous reference to women's promiscuity while their husbands were whisked away by the Crusades. Cheeky women.

That said, something about them clearly captivated cultural attention. Into the sixteenth century, we can see satirical illustra-

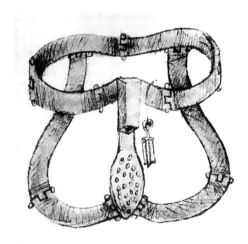

The illustration from Kyeser's manuscript, *Bellifortis*, of a chastity belt that appears notably uncomfortable and unwieldy.

tions of these devices, along with the figure of the cuckold. Naked wives are commonly depicted wearing them in bed while their husbands bid them adieu—all the while at least one man hides in the corner of the room holding a replica of the husband's key. These images played into the popular depiction of the foolish cuckold that fascinated the public at the time. Often, the husband is drawn with animal ears or horns growing out of his head.

In one illustration, now held in the British Museum, a husband with donkey-like ears attached to his hat retrieves the key from his wife. The ears closely resemble the hat of the fool at his feet, who is unsuccessfully attempting to trap fleas inside a basket. Try as he may, the husband, just like the fool, is unlikely to prevent his creature from flying away. Indeed, two men are hiding in the shadows behind the bed, and the only thing that manages to catch the light is the key in one of their hands. As Sarah Laskow has summarized Classen's argument, "male fear" was the ingredient that kept the story of this device alive:

> Even in the 1500s, no one took the idea of locked-up metal underwear very seriously as an effective anti-sex device. When chastity belts were depicted, it was in the Renaissance equivalent of Robin Hood: Men in Tights—and the audiences for those pieces of art probably thought the idea of a metal chastity belt just as giggle-worthy as late 20th-century teenagers did.
>
> This idea of the untamable wife and the humiliated husband clearly tickled an area of our fancy. In the nineteenth century, we decided to finally bring these belts into existence. As the British Museum bluntly states: "It is probable that the great majority of examples now existing were made in the eighteenth and nineteenth centuries as curiosities for the prurient, or as jokes for the tasteless." The Victorian era became obsessed with the idea of the Dark Ages as a barbarous and cruel time. It could well be the case that fake belts were created to pass off as authentic devices from the period. If so, they were successful—many contemporary museums displayed these belts as "medieval artifacts" until fairly recently, when the likes of Classen began to call their authenticity into question.

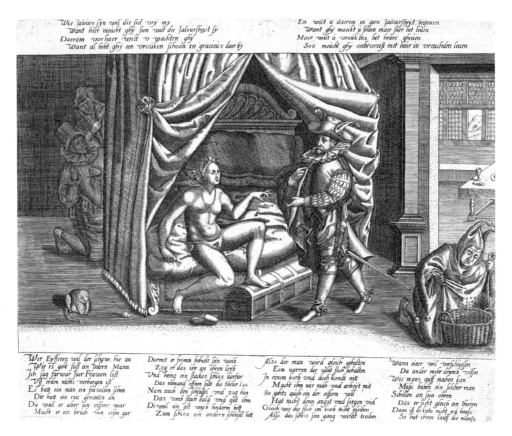

This satirical sixteenth-century print by Heinrich Wirrich, currently housed in the British Museum, humorously portrays a chastity belt in use.

It is also likely, however, that some models may have been created to finally fulfill the fantasies they had awakened, particularly as production methods were now up to the task of doing so inexpensively. What started as a theological allegory and evolved into a satirical joke now emerges as an IRL fantasy. Pornography holds more than just the power to arouse, it also has the power to bring things to life—a topic we shall discuss with our dessert.

For now, it is enough to offer this comfort: in case you've ever been made to feel bad about it, just know that your little penis cage is rooted in history.

By exploring these rooms tonight, I hope that the half of you who have admitted to having experienced some kind of kinky desire finally see yourselves represented.

Indeed, the reality is that we may number much higher. We all know there can be considerable bias affecting large studies, as people are less likely to admit to desires and behaviors that are generally considered shameful or irregular. Imagine how much higher this statistic may climb once this conversation becomes more mainstream.

Social media has opened up the possibility of change. TikTok, Instagram, and You-Tube have exposed billions of people to new and exciting ideas and brought awareness about kinks and fetishes into the wider world. In fact, #KinkTok is one of the most popular hashtags on TikTok. At the time of writing, it has received over twelve billion views. For many people, this is the first time they have been exposed to others speaking and educating on this sexual practice. TikTok has become a place of self-discovery, with many people claiming they have realized (or found the words to describe) their sexual desires and orientation by using the app. There are reasonable concerns with this kind of immediate, unevenly regulated access to sex-related content on a public app, but as my experiences with online games in primary school prove, that's true for nearly everything on the internet. As well as continuing to foster safer virtual environments, I also believe keeping this kind of content on these platforms caters to the need for broad access, good education, and healthy conversation.

There was another commonality in the studies that found half of the population to be a little bit kinky—and that was the huge amount of respondents who emphasized the need for community and education. These were the factors that helped them fight back feelings of loneliness, anxiety, and alienation when it came to their desires. Instead, they experienced acceptance, empowerment, and understanding.

If we utilize these advances to their full potential, we could improve the dialogue surrounding kinky sexuality, providing a safer environment, greater sexual freedom, more understanding about our desires—and, hey, maybe even better sex! The spiking interest in these topics provides an opportunity to change our relationship to kinks and fetishes, to get rid of shame. That all starts with reconsidering the way we tell history.

#LearnOnTikTok, at the time of writing, has received over five hundred billion views. These numbers speak for themselves. Young people especially want to learn and find community on digital platforms. However, if we are going to change the narrative, we have to talk about gender, sex, and identity in a way that is uninhibited, vulnerable, and real. I try to educate people about the history of sex from a place of passion and authenticity. I try to speak about what I have learned and what I have experienced in a way that is not held back by cultural stigmas of shame and repulsion.

I would like to envision a time when kinks and fetishes are not considered radical to talk about: a time when we recognize the universality *and* diversity of sex as an experience, as a form of play, as a place of empathy. A time when we can stop treating the act that connects us all as a reason for so much division. It all comes from finally talking about these parts of who we are, and who we've always been. If we can tell a story of history in which we finally write these stories back into the pages, we can see how kinks and fetishes have always played their part—even in the lives of our most esteemed figures.

I hope by now it goes without saying that this sexual liberation is no one-way, linear journey. History is an endless stream, ebbing and flowing, alternately propelling us forward and pulling us backward.

There is a kind of beauty in living in paradox, in (dare I say it?) encompassing and celebrating many shades of gray. While liberation and destigmatization are political and social goods, so many of our desires are for the taboo, the forbidden fruit. Can we ever be completely sexually liberated—and is that even something that would be desirable? If we were to normalize the desires and behaviors before us tonight, surely a new range would appear. Part of the appeal of kinks and fetishes is the sense of existing and indeed reveling in deviance. It feels really good to be a little bit bad. It is a needed escape, a release, from the rules of propriety we follow in the real world every single day. I think this is why nearly every practiced kinkster I know is a good, ethically motivated person. They have found their safe release from the constraints of polite society—a relief every human needs—and can enjoy the taboo in a safe, consensual environment. They have no need to misbehave in their day-to-day lives. Maybe if we were all more like kinksters, the world would be a better place.

Ah, there is the bell. It is time for us to enjoy our final course. Come, Rousseau and Lewis, Berkley and Shakespeare. Let us put away our whips and our horns, our leather paddles and our chastity belts. The same goes for those who have snuck away to the library. Take your books with you, if you can't bring yourself to put them down. I'm sure they will be fantastic inspiration for our next conversation.

The only soul left outside the dining room is the cat, who has fallen asleep by the library fire. She is lying on something, a slumbering dragon protecting its treasure. Slide it out so we can see what it has to say.

Well, it seems that we are familiar with its contents already. I assure you, dear cat, there was nothing to worry about. We will return it to its rightful owner.

Wouldn't it be lovely to think that someday, when someone else finds Joyce's letters, they won't think he was a little bit freaky—they will instead think that he was a little bit human?

THE PORN KINK

We have now reached everyone's favorite course—dessert. The table is filled with figs, pomegranates, chocolates, and tarts. The wine continues to flow as coffee and tea are being served. What a transformation since the beginning of the evening! Masters and Johnson are up on the table performing a tango while Mozart plays a dirty ditty. Joyce has picked a fight with Freud, crying, "Deal with him, Hemingway! Deal with him!" Mistress Berkley is keeping Rousseau well amused in the hall, where as many guests as possible can watch, and Lewis is politely waiting his turn. Stein has lit up a cigar with Alfred Kinsey and is explaining the erotic connotations of the art hanging on the wall. The room is alight with conversation, with passionate debates across tables and whispered observations in corners. If you listen closely, you can tune in to each of their worlds in turn, as ideas are shared and opinions loudly proclaimed. If you sit back and listen to them all, it is music: hundreds of conversations meeting and clashing in an awe-inspiring, chaotic harmony. This is the sound of a good dinner party.

Have you had a moment to look at the books brought in from the library? Disreputable tomes for a dinner table, and I believe this lot only brought them in to look at the pictures: *Dangerous Liaisons*, *Justine*, *Venus in Furs*,* and *Story of O*. All have caused a variety of scandals—which reminds me of my final topic for the night.

Picture this scenario, dear friends: It's 1:35 p.m. The day thus far has been filled with email pings, takeaway coffee, and this-could-have-been-an-email-

---

* Originally *Les Liaisons Dangereuses* (1782), *Justine, ou Les Malheurs de la Vertu* (1791), and *Venus im Pelz* (1870).

style Zoom calls. The novelty of working from home wore off months ago, and it is now one long monotonous *Groundhog Day* of switched-off cameras and sweatpants. Though there is *one* thing that's not too bad about it all . . . one ritual that makes the day somewhat bearable, if only momentarily. You shut the laptop, slither to the next room, plonk yourself on the bed (thank god for those sweatpants), and pull out your phone. Do Not Disturb mode on (why are people sending emails over the lunch hour, anyway?). Incognito mode on. And just like that, you enjoy three minutes of sexual pleasure, allowing yourself to forget about the workday and the depressing drama of the outside world.

It's really no wonder that pornography views rose so drastically over the course of the pandemic. Confined to the house 24-7 with increased dependence upon the internet and smartphones is a logical recipe for more me-time indulgence. Data reports from 2020 make it clear that the cities in lockdown were making the best possible use of their time. Pornhub reported that in the first three months of 2020, 80 percent of Australian traffic to their site came from three states in lockdown: New South Wales (31.6 percent), Victoria (27.1 percent), and Queensland (20.6 percent). Perhaps due to our extended time in lockdown, Australia, by the following year, ranked seventh on the list of countries who most frequently visit Pornhub. If that wasn't enough to make you feel like a proud Australian, these statistics also show that Aussies on average last longer than any other country. The average person spends a total of nine minutes and seven seconds on Pornhub, while Aussies take gold with a whopping nine minutes and twenty-four seconds. (Every second counts.)

While we've all been fanning our own flames, this increased collective self-loving behavior has also oxygenated an ongoing discussion about the effects, positive and negative, of our cultural consumption of pornography. This conversation is far from new, yet we haven't come to any set conclusion as to: Is pornography dangerous? Will watching it decrease our sex drives? Does it glorify violence? Can we find a way to consume it ethically?

This is not a recent debate; we have been embroiled in it for hundreds of years. Pornography has a rich and complex history, one with roots (go on, guess!) all the way back in the ancient world. By looking back at the various cultural—and sometimes, spiritual—roles that pornography as we would now classify it has played, we can begin to find the answers to our burning questions about this popular genre.

Prior to the pandemic, pornography was already a hot topic of research, funded and referred to rather liberally as a rapidly growing public health concern. Shocking reports from the 2000s showed that rates of lifetime exposure to pornography were 73 to 93 percent for adolescent boys and 11 to 62 percent for adolescent girls in Australia. Technology has been much blamed. The ease of access to the internet, computers, and smartphones led to a new era of free pornography. Younger millennials were a particular point of interest. What impact would it have on the developing human brain to be able to access footage of sexual activities whenever an urge arose—or perhaps, more concerning, even when it didn't, when one stumbled upon it? The main concern was that this takes the power of education away from the school or family home, giving it all to the smartphone, already viewed with suspicion.

A 2017 Australian study found that the median age for viewing pornography for the first time was thirteen years of age for male respondents and sixteen years for female ones. With time now to analyze the impact of this early and ongoing exposure, it was determined that more frequent pornography viewing was associated with male gender, younger age, higher education, nonheterosexual identity, ever having had anal intercourse, and recent mental health problems, a notably extensive and rather vague list of outcomes, with no clear indication of which factor impacted which or to what extent. As seems to be the case with most studies examining the potentially negative "public health impact," the paper comes to the conclusion that further research is needed—a phrase all too familiar to those who have come into contact with the academic world. But rather than awaiting the creation of more deviants, unwittingly informed by unchecked exposure to their phones, perhaps it would be more rewarding for us to look back through pornography's long and rich history.

A Portrait of the Artist
Using One Hand

While pornography has been defined as a genre only since (wait for it) the eighteenth century, its origins date back to the ancient world. Many ancient Egyptian religious myths, which were told in stories or depicted in art, revolve heavily around sexual themes. The tales of their gods and goddesses really read like one long Wattpad story.

Egyptian mythology all starts with the god Atum, who wanks the world into existence. From his sacred semen came the air god, Shu, and the moisture goddess, fittingly named Tefnut.

> *Atum created by his masturbation in Heliopolis. He put his phallus in his fist, to*
> *excite desire thereby. The twins were born, Shu and Tefnut.*

Horniness was as hereditary as holiness in this family. The grandchildren, Geb, the god of the earth, and Nut (fittingly, once again), goddess of the sky, would become the most active hornbags that the universe had seen to date (and yes, they were twins). The two were so busy making love all the time that party pooper grandpa Atum finally had enough. He separated them, trampled Geb, forming the earth, and lifted Nut up high, forming the sky. What grumpy Gramps hadn't anticipated was his grandchildren's flexibility when it came to matters of lust—flexibility being the key word, as Geb is often depicted performing fellatio on himself in acrobatic positions. Perhaps *he* was the one who donated that rib to Eve . . .

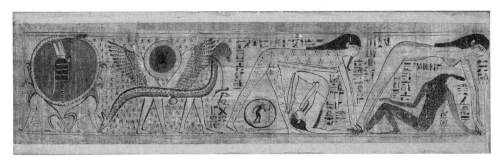

This illustration from the Book of the Dead of Henuttawy shows Geb putting his newfound flexibility to good use.

While sentenced to the sky, Nut would give birth to the children conceived during her love affair with her twin brother. These children were sure to do their family proud. Indeed, one of the oldest depictions of oral sex comes from their tale—talk about a legacy! Osiris married his sister, Isis, and gained the hatred of his brother, Set. Osiris was the god of order, and Set was the god of chaos, and to fulfill his dream of universal chaos, Set orchestrated the murder of his brother and severed his body into fourteen pieces. Isis was, understandably, not too happy about her husband being chopped up like sashimi. She set out in search of the pieces . . . But there was one pretty crucial part still missing, because in a performance of true alpha masculinity, Set had chopped his brother's dick off and thrown it to the fishes. (Plutarch claimed this is why eating fish is taboo in Egypt—you didn't want to be chomping down on a tuna sandwich only to find you'd eaten your favorite god's willy.) As you may remember from earlier in the evening, Isis was forced to call upon her artistic abilities, molding a penis out of mud and attaching it to the reassembled body. The goddess of magic then proceeded to perform one hell of a blow job, literally blowing her brother back to life.

You would really think the story would end here, as all good stories should, with one final, magical gobby. Not so. These horny deities would then take it all one step further. Cue the Semen Wars. Looking to avenge his father and his fish-food penis, Horus ended up in a series of peculiar battles with Set, which became exceedingly bizarre once they took their fight into the bedroom. The events are detailed in the Chester Beatty Papyrus I:

> Now afterward, [at] evening time, bed was prepared for them, and they both lay down. But during the night, Set caused his phallus to become stiff and inserted it between Horus's thighs. Then Horus placed his hands between his thighs and received Set's semen. Horus went to tell his mother Isis: "Help me, Isis, my mother, come and see what Set has done to me." And he opened his hand[s] and let her see Set's semen. She let out a loud shriek, seized the copper [knife], cut off his hand[s] that were equivalent. Then she fetched some fragrant ointment and applied it to Horus's phallus. She caused it to become stiff and inserted it into a pot, and he caused his semen to flow down into it.

This may seem like an overreaction on Isis's part, but we must understand that for Horus to be covered in the semen of another man was defilement and degradation. Cutting off his hands was the only way to remove the evidence that this act had taken place. Isis takes the pot of her son's semen to her brother's house (note, not the one who is also her husband) and there inquires with the gardener about which vegetables Set likes to eat. In the weirdest part of the story, it is declared that *lettuce* is Set's favorite food, so Isis then pours her son's semen on Set's illogically beloved meal, which he unwittingly consumes.

Lettuce was actually considered an aphrodisiac in ancient Egypt and was the favored food of the fertility god, Min, as well. We have Horus's semen to thank for this. As you may have noticed, a white substance oozes out when you cut a lettuce leaf in half. And that, my friend, was thought to be leftover god cum.

In comparison to the wild stories of the sexual proclivities of their gods, most ancient Egyptian art is tame. One reason for this is that sex was seen as an unremarkable activity. As archaeologist Charlotte Booth has remarked, "Many common Egyptian activities, like childbirth and mummification, were not considered interesting enough to be recorded. . . . Sex was on a par with eating, sleeping and defecating and was linked to all aspects of life." The artistic conventions of the time held that key parts of the body and face had to be clearly depicted for the deceased to get a chance to use their body in the afterlife. This is why art thought to depict people kissing—such as in the case of the two men, Niankhkhnum and Khnumhotep, whom we discussed earlier—will come no closer than nose-to-nose.

This is not to say that there are no erotic paintings from the period—just that they all have beautiful side profiles. The most renowned erotic art is the Turin Erotic Papyrus, dated to around 1150 BCE. Though it was known to Egyptologists from the 1820s, it was only made public in the 1970s. Fragments discovered in the Egyptian Museum in Turin, Italy, only hint at what the full version would have been. Measuring over 2.5 meters, this ancient scroll-painting contains twelve distinct erotic pictures. While much of the work has unfortunately been damaged over time, it is still possible to make out some of the imagery, such as the ginormous genitalia of the men, the incredible flexibility of the women, the use of vases and chariots to aid erotic acts, and, of course, a monkey.

There has been considerable speculation surrounding the purpose of this scroll. Is it the ancient version of *Penthouse*? Did it have some kind of religious purpose, akin to the semen battles and magic blow jobs of the gods? Or could it have been political critique? This final reasoning is the most convincing. The pornographic illustrations on the "Turin Satirical-Erotic Papyrus" could have been intended as social commentary on class differences. Just like many of the political cartoons found in newspapers today, unflattering caricatures were a popular way to deliver punchy satire in ancient Egypt. Despite their enormous schlongs, the men in these pictures do not conform to the typical standard of beauty of the time. It has therefore been suggested that artists could have been mocking lower-class citizens so their "superiors" could laugh at the animal-like ways of the poor. Conversely, it could have been made with the intention of mocking those members of the aristocracy, condemning their excessive, morally corrupt behaviors. Who knew that pornography could be such a powerful political tool?

To answer that question strategically posed to myself: French pamphleteers during the revolution! What does the French Revolution have to do with pornography, I hear you say. Well, practically everything.

My own research traces an aesthetic of the erotic in eighteenth-century literature, because works of this time were *exploding* with sexual connotations and erotic desire. It's no exaggeration to say that the emergence of pornography as a literary genre changed the course of our sexual history. We underestimate just how much power pornography has had (and continues to have) in not only reflecting but *shaping* society, and pornographic writings were one of the primary influences over revolutionary passions in the French general public.

Shocking erotic depictions of the French aristocracy in pornographic pamphlets, plays, and more helped to generate widespread hatred and disdain for them. As perfectly summarized by academic Lynn Hunt, "Politically motivated pornography helped to bring about the Revolution by undermining the legitimacy of the ancien régime as a social and political system." Noble women were depicted as lesbians (*shock!*), the king was depicted as a cuckold (*horror!*), and all the royal court was depicted to partake in regular group orgies (*scandal!*).

Marie Antoinette was the most popular subject of these attacks. On a list of erotic pamphlets confiscated by Parisian police in 1790–1791, those featuring Marie Antoinette were the two most popular—"Vie privée, libertine, et scandaleuse de Marie-Antoinette," with eighty-eight confiscated copies, and "La Messaline française," with eighty-one. While Marie Antoinette was portrayed as a prolific libertine, Louis XVI was her foolish cuckold. In the opera *L'Autrichienne en goguettes, ou l'orgie royale* (1789), Charles X pleasures both Marie Antoinette and the Duchess of Polignac while Louis XVI sleeps on a couch. Who says operas are boring?

The scandalous depictions succeeded in making these authority figures utterly ridiculous to the public eye. These kinds of publications were not too dissimilar to modern gossip magazines. There were generally published under the guise of truth, as real stories from the courts that had made it out via an anonymous person of importance—the historical version of "You just have to believe me, OK?" After a time, it didn't matter if these stories were fact or fiction, as their sustained repetition caused them to take on a reality of their own. Keep in mind as well that the printing press, and more widespread literacy, was still new. There wasn't the same kind of emphasis as there is today on fact-checking or verifying claims (though an argument could well be made that we still care too little about this today). It was all clickbait headlines, and they crept into people's subconscious minds.

When the revolution finally came about, the inspiration for the acts of sexual violence committed against aristocrats can be found in the more popular pornographic pamphlets. No slander is more powerful than sexual slander.

Revenge porn, which involves the nonconsensual sharing of explicit images or videos, has become a particularly insidious form of this slander in the digital age. Unlike the localized examples from history, revenge porn can reach a global audience, causing irreparable harm to the victim's reputation and well-being. Similar to the anonymous pamphlets of the past, the anonymity and distance provided by the internet can make it difficult for victims to seek justice and hold perpetrators accountable. While sexual slander has a long history, the digital age has brought new and alarming dimensions.

The erotic can be harnessed not only to arouse our bodies and imaginations in both positive and negative ways, but to sway our social and political beliefs. It's no wonder, then, that sex is used so frequently in advertising. I strongly believe that exploring the political role pornography has played throughout history means we can be more conscious consumers of all erotic media. When we're in a heightened state of arousal, we make ourselves vulnerable, and this in turn makes us susceptible and malleable. Sex researcher Dr. Justin Lehmiller has observed that what we view during orgasm can shape our future fantasies, as we come to relate this image with the experienced feeling of pleasure. That is a considerable amount of power, especially in politically charged hands.

A Short History of
Erotic Literature

Or, The Awankening

I f we are going to become more conscious consumers of pornography, we first need
to define exactly what it is. How do we decide what's porn and what isn't? Does it
only constitute videos of one or more people performing sexual acts? Do written
works, like *Fifty Shades of Grey*, classify as porn? And what about random images, such
as erotic advertisements, that just happen to turn some people on? The fact is, "pornography" looks different to everyone. While we can, and should, have a formal definition for the sake of clear communication, it won't cover all the media or the way these
evolve over time. Take, for example, this definition of pornography as Peter Wagner
saw it functioning in the eighteenth century:

> *I would define eighteenth-century pornography as the written or visual pre-
> sentation in a realistic form of any genital or sexual behaviour with a deliber-
> ate violation of existing and widely accepted moral and social taboos.*

While pornography today can certainly cross into the realm of taboo, it is unlikely
that many of us would see this aspect as intrinsic to its definition as a genre. Conversely, as we have seen, pornography in the eighteenth century was often politically

motivated, used to critique social and moral attitudes. While we have a range of erotic art and literature dating back to the ancient world that we now classify as pornography, this was not even considered as a distinctly separate category until the early nineteenth century. What's more, we can once again see it was only categorized and given a name in an effort to *police* a trend in written and visual media that used the shock factor of sex as a way to criticize religious and political authorities. This wasn't just a genre for horny storytelling, this was a "cultural battle zone."

If we are going to sit here discussing pornography, then there really is someone you must meet. Are you here, Aretino? Leave the cook alone and come and meet our guest! Pietro Aretino (1492–1556) is recognized as one of the forefathers of pornography as a literary genre. Pietro was an Italian writer best known in his time for being an outspoken critic of the authorities. He can be described as a deviant queer figure, too, having proudly declared himself a sodomite, who claimed in a letter to have only "temporarily switched from boys to girls" in 1524 after he'd "fallen in love with a female cook." He was such an influential figure in the history of pornography that one of his works, best known now as *Aretino's Postures*, is a defining work for the entire genre.

Marcantonio Raimondi (alongside the Renaissance master Raphael) turned erotic paintings by Giulio Romano into sixteen engravings of sexual positions. Look, someone has been kind enough to leave us a copy here on the table. This publication was released in 1523, titled *I Modi* (*The Ways*), though perhaps it's best known as *The Sixteen Pleasures*. The Catholic Church was far from amused. Pope Clement VII immediately ordered the destruction of all copies of this work and the imprisonment of Raimondi.

However, Aretino had a different opinion of the whole endeavor. Fascinated with the work, he paid a trip to Romano (who had not been informed that his paintings were being turned into engravings). Inspired by the work of the original images, Aretino composed sixteen erotic sonnets to accompany them—works explicit enough to make us blush today. By 1527, *I Modi* would go to print a second time, now including both the illustrations and accompanying sonnets. Many scholars mark this as the first time erotic writing and images were published together for the sole purpose of arousing the reader. (It should also be mentioned that Aretino secured Raimondi's release from prison—he didn't leave his brother hanging.)

The destruction of this publication was quickly ordered, but distributors appeared better prepared this time. While none of the original engravings exist, enough must have escaped the clutches of the Catholic Church that the publication continued to be copied frequently, ensuring its survival in various forms. From its English translations, *I Modi* received the name that it is commonly known as today, *Aretino's Postures*.

Aretino's influence did not stop here. He penned a second work that heavily influenced the future of pornography as a genre, *Ragionamenti* (1534, 1536), a dramatic dialogue between an experienced sex worker and her novice counterpart. This dialogue provided a kind of sex education, both fictionally for the young woman and practically for the reader. Aretino's work offered an instructional guide to how sex should be spoken about by society. He advocated for doing away with tiptoeing around the subject, and instead start calling a spade a spade. Listen to him now.

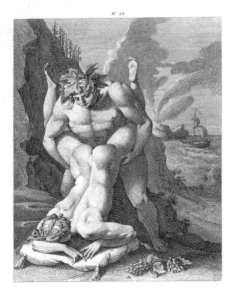

BACHUS ET ARIANE.

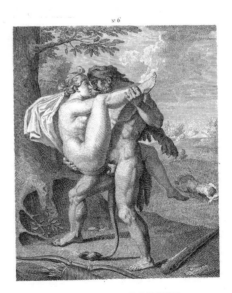

HERCULE ET DEJANIRE

Engravings from Agostino Carracci's *The Aretin or Collection of Erotic Postures*, printed in Paris in 1798, which allude to *I Modi*.

Nº 18.

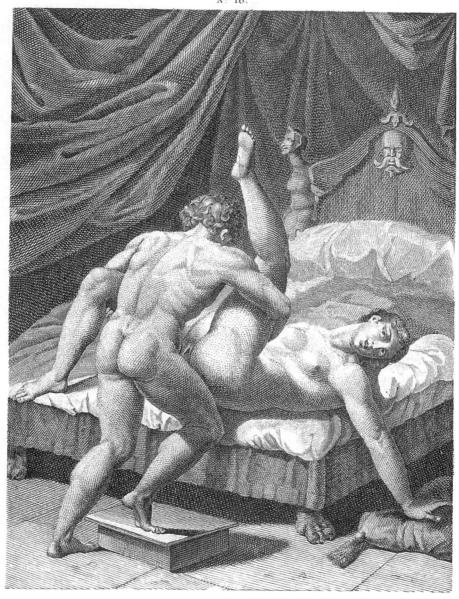

ALCIBIADE ET GLYCERE

Oh, I meant to tell you and then I forgot: Speak plainly and say "fuck," "prick,"
"cunt" and "ass" if you want anyone except the scholars at the University of
Rome to understand you . . . why don't you say it straight out and stop going
about on tiptoes? Why don't you say yes when you mean yes and no when you
mean no—or else keep it to yourself?

Five hundred years later, a lot of Aretino's work continues to ring true.

Dialogue between an experienced and novice sex worker became a popular trope in the genre that would later be called "pornography." In fact, it inspired the work that is now considered the first pornographic novel, *Memoirs of a Woman of Pleasure* (otherwise known as *Fanny Hill*) by John Cleland (1749). We have already brought this book out once tonight. Shall we pass it around again?

When this novel was released it shook the world—literally. On March 8, 1750, an expurgated version was released, the same day a devastating earthquake struck London, destroying treasured buildings and leaving the public alarmed. Authorities could not believe these two events were unrelated, the Bishop Sherlock declaring that the publication of the book—"the lewdest thing I ever saw"—had been enough to bring down the wrath of God. *Memoirs* had already been published in two parts the year before, and Cleland was brought to prosecution for violating obscenity statutes. Even he refused to vindicate his actions in penning this notorious book, stating before the court it was "a Book I disdain to defend, and wish, from the bottom of my Soul, buried and forgot."

My deepest apologies to Cleland, but I have never been one who cared much for the Do Not Disturb sign.

The novel consists of two letters, supposedly written by Fanny Hill, who exposes all the "scandalous stages of [her] life" to an unnamed correspondent. These salacious letters took the world by storm—*Memoirs* became a bestseller in eighteenth-century Europe and has virtually never been out of print since. The book's influence on the world of literature is undeniable, as many consider it to be "the first original prose pornography."

There is something so seductive and exciting about being privy to a conversation of which you were not meant to be part, a fact that erotic writers of the eighteenth century knew well. A plethora of literature was released at the time that pretended (sometimes to the point of actually duping the reader) to be written by the hand of women confessing their scandalous stories or secrets to their friends. Sometimes, the author would say that they had uncovered these letters in the drawers of well-known women, and believed it was their social duty to bring such sinful confessions to light.*

Memoirs plays into this trope, though Cleland did not hide the fact of his authorship. The erotic novel is written in the form of two lengthy letters to an unnamed confidante of Fanny's. In these letters, she recounts her salacious journey from a young, naive country girl to a woman who has been educated in the world of pleasures through her profession as a sex worker. She claims her letters contain nothing but the "stark, naked truth" and endeavors to write her tale with the same liberty with which she lived it.

But what was it that made *Memoirs* in particular so scandalous?

This novel still takes new readers by surprise with its illicit and, in places, progressive content. Fanny's introduction to the world of pleasure begins with a queer encounter—the roaming hands of her bedmate, Phoebe. And this is far from the only homoerotic encounter—Fanny and her follow sex workers in their women-run brothel freely share kisses and caresses.

In a time dominated by conversation on "how to find the clitoris," modern readers may be shocked by Cleland's understanding of the female body. He mentions such detail as the swelling that occurs in her "tender parts" following vigorous consummation, and notes how a pillow can be placed underneath the woman's back to enhance the experience for both parties in heterosexual missionary. All this said, the novel can hardly be thought physiologically accurate—Fanny does manage to live a libertine life in London without one unwanted pregnancy, disease, or period.

However, it was not this or even the whipping scenes, which we spoke about earlier, that brought Cleland to prosecution. It was the inclusion of a homoerotic scene between two men. Fanny spies on two men who have taken up lodgings in a room next to her. Witnessing the act of anal sex shocks her so much she falls unconscious on the

---

* *Exhibition of Female Flagellants* proudly displays on its title page that it has simply recounted stories "from authentic anecdotes, French and English, found in a Lady's Cabinet" and that the editor has done so to prove "from indubitable facts, that a number of ladies take a secret pleasure, in whipping their own." Basically, a fantastic excuse to detail some queer sadomasochistic fantasies.

floor. Out of all the sexual acts that Fanny observes, this is the only one that she cannot comprehend. Despite the novel's condemnation of the act, its mere inclusion was enough for it to be considered an affront to polite society.

Sex acts between men, in particular sodomy, were becoming criminalized at the time that Cleland was writing. While sodomy had technically been illegal in Europe prior to the eighteenth century, this period saw the introduction of far more severe forms of prosecution—and undoubtedly a higher level of male anxiety as a result. *Memoirs* was most likely written by a homosexual author at a time of growing homophobia. While writers such as Aretino could wear their sexualities as a "pendant around our necks as we wear a badge in our caps," Cleland was at far greater risk of serious consequences.

There is convincing evidence for the likelihood of Cleland's homosexual desire. In 1781, the antiquary Josiah Beckwith wrote that Cleland unfortunately "pass[ed] under the Censure of being a Sodomite, as he now does, and in Consequence thereof Persons of Character decline visiting him, or cultivating his Acquaintance." Further biographical details, such as a rumored offense during his schooling years and his unmarried status, have led some scholars to infer Cleland's homosexuality—his relationship with Thomas Cannon was a matter of particular conjecture. Hal Gladfelder has noted the potential implications of Cleland's friendship with the author of *Ancient and Modern Pederasty Investigated and Exemplify'd*, which he considers the earliest surviving published defense of homosexuality in English. Gladfelder states, "It's no coincidence that they simultaneously produced the only two explicit accounts of male same-sex desire in English before the late nineteenth century, published just a month apart."

So pornography—a genre now often associated with heteronormative depictions of sexuality—was actually popularized as a genre by two (likely) queer men who wrote through the eyes of female sex workers. Over the following centuries, the genre transformed from its original vision as a socially disruptive and conversational art form. Today, pornographers are far more motivated by helping people get a hard-on than by the chance to take down a corrupt regime.

The term *pornography* would not appear in the *Oxford English Dictionary* until 1857. It found its origins slightly earlier as the French term *le pornographe*, which referred to writings on prostitution and other "obscene" matters. It is defined by the *Oxford En-*

glish Dictionary (finally!) as "printed or visual material containing the explicit description or display of sexual organs or activity, intended to stimulate sexual excitement." This definition allows for a wide scope of what we can classify as pornography.

The first time I ever masturbated with the aid of "visual material" was in ye olde days of YouTube to a homemade video of Barbie dolls. Yep. I was really quite young at the time, and had no idea what masturbating even was—back then it was just a pleasant, harmless tingling feeling that happened when you rubbed down there. What I wasn't counting on, in my journey to understand my body, was that a video of Barbie in her Dreamhouse doing the splits with Ken could set these feelings off. A shitty homemade video of Ken and Barbie smushing their faces together and then lingering spread-eagle on the bed got my starter engines running, apparently.

I was (and am) as shocked as you are. I hadn't gone out of my way to find this video. It was just . . . there . . . down a YouTube hole: a video considered tame enough to even be on their more stringently censored platform of the time. It was simply two plastic dolls smashing into each other.

Looking back at this truly bizarre sexual awakening, I have many questions. (Just *why?* encompasses most of them.) Perhaps the most important one for our purposes would be whether or not this video classifies as pornography.

"Visual material," check.

Containing the "explicit description or display of sexual organs" . . . "Sexual organs" is a stretch, but I think we can at least classify the gyration of plastic limbs as sexual behavior.

"Intended to stimulate sexual excitement." Well, it's hard to know what on earth, exactly, *Imabarbiegirl69* hoped to achieve in making this video, but we can assume that sexual excitement was part of it. So did they, incidentally, create a porno in the Barbie Dreamhouse?

When it comes to defining pornography, intention for use is a critical factor. This definition came to the forefront of a criminal case in Massachusetts, *Commonwealth v. Rex*, 469 Mass. 36 (2014), which investigated the possession of nude photographs of children by a convicted sex offender. To the outrage of many, it was finally ruled that these photographs did not classify as child pornography because of the *intention* behind them. These photographs had been published in *National Geographic* magazines, sociology textbooks, and nudist magazines. They could not, as a result, fulfill this criterion for the definition of pornography. The justices reported:

> *The visibility of the children's genitals is merely an inherent aspect of the fact that they are naked. There is nothing remotely sexual, either explicitly or implicitly, in any of the photocopies. The demeanor, facial expressions, and body language of the children suggest nothing inappropriate.*

There was a huge amount of backlash to this decision, and the ruling triggered a public conversation about what was more crucial when defining pornography—the intention of the creator or of the consumer? There is no clear-cut answer. It becomes even harder to answer when keeping in mind that what pornography looks like varies so greatly from person to person. What turns one person on may seem harmless and silly to someone else, and a source of genuine alarm to a third person.

What we need to hold in mind is the time and place in which that piece of media exists. Culture has an immeasurable impact on our ethics as well as our conceptions of the erotic. This can be readily evidenced from the different ideas of what we consider sexy.

Their Eyes Were Watching Hentai

C ontrary to popular belief, eroticized parts of the human body—such as boobs or buttocks—may not *naturally* arouse us. Studies have found that our arousal and fetishized interest in these body parts may be culturally conditioned, a line of thought influenced by the work of anthropologist Clellan S. Ford and ethologist Frank A. Beach. Their 1951 publication, *Patterns of Sexual Behavior*, compared information about sexual desire and behavior from 191 different cultures (47 from Oceania, 28 from Eurasia, 33 from Africa, 57 from North America, and 26 from South America). One of the most fascinating finds is the different ways members of these cultures thought about and reacted to female breasts.

Now, sexual interest in breasts is a well recognized fact in Western cultures today; a study of Belgium's population declared that 86.7 percent of men have this particular fetish interest. Yet Ford and Beach's study found that this was far from the case across all cultures. In fact, out of the 191 cultures they investigated, breasts were thought of as sexually stimulating to men in only 13. Even among those, there was little agreement regarding which kind of breasts are attractive. Nine had a preference for larger breasts, while the other four were divided between long, erect, and circular breasts. Another inconsistency is that only 13 cultures in this study claimed that stimulation of the breasts provided important foreplay—however, only three of these were among the cultures that found the sight of breasts arousing. While this study is outdated now, it has provided invaluable insight into the role cultural factors can play in the creation of our sexual desires. Milkshakes do not, in fact, bring all boys to the yard.

This logic helps to explain why, in many ancient cultures, depictions of genitals could be used as benign decoration throughout cities. If you've visited the surviving sites of ancient Rome, you may have noticed many doodles of doodles, especially in the remains of Pompeii. In 79 BCE, this ancient Roman city was buried in the ash of Mount Vesuvius, a volcano located in Italy's Gulf of Naples. This tragedy resulted in the preservation of many artifacts—as well as the bodies of over a thousand city inhabitants—providing us unique access to this ancient world.

Pompeii is infamous in our cultural memory as a place of licentiousness and surprising liberality. Tourists continue to flock to the ruins of this once vibrant city, often finding themselves giggling over the number of stone phalluses carved into the remaining pavement and walls, some hanging invitingly above doorways and ovens. These establishments were popular in Pompeii: sex work was not only legal, it was regarded as the social norm for men (and, in some rare cases, wealthier women) to frequent such establishments.

Sexuality and sexual behavior in ancient Rome were not bound by the same shameful stigmas we know today. Regarded no differently than other bodily behaviors, sex came with its own social rules on the acceptable ways of engagement. This all being said, sex work of the time was intricately tied to slavery. A census suggested that by 3000 BCE, there were over thirty-two thousand sex workers operating throughout Rome.

The industry was one the most lucrative sources of revenue for the Roman Empire, and Rome became known as the ancient capital of sex work. During his reign, the emperor Caligula implemented a notorious tax on sex-work services, commonly known as the "imperial tax," in which a portion of the fee paid by customers to the sex workers was collected and deposited into the state treasury. The tax law was later upheld by Severus Alexander when he assumed power, but the collected funds were instead directed toward the maintenance of public buildings. The economics of brothels were heavily influenced by legal and tax regulations such as these.

The majority of these workers would have been enslaved women, a smaller percentage of enslaved men, and an even smaller number who were freed slaves or poor freeborn women. The conditions of their brothels were nothing to be envied, some quarters being no better than concrete cells without windows. Enslaved workers were cut off from the rest of the world, living solely within these premises with only their basic needs provided for.

One brothel in the city of Pompeii remains open for customers today—tourists only, rather than the clientele for whom it was intended. The Lupanar of Pompeii began to be excavated in 1862. This two-story establishment has been of particular interest to

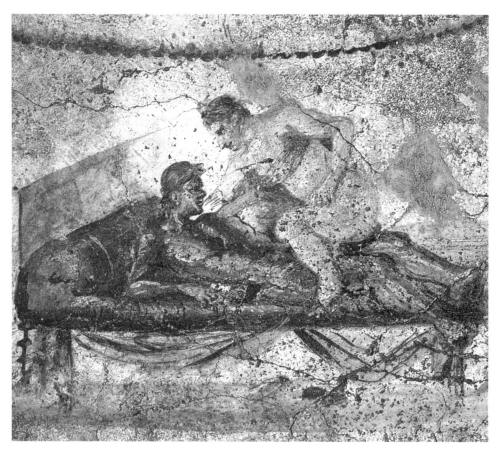

In the Lupanar brothel of Pompeii, a wall painting features a woman, believed to be a sex worker, in the act with a client.

the curious traveler due to the erotic and humorous graffiti and artwork inside. Over 150 of the scrawls on the walls have now been translated for the public's enjoyment: including *Hic ego puellas multas futui* ("Here many girls poked") and *Felix bene futuis* ("Lucky guy, you get a good fuck"). The art throughout is equally engaging, putting to rest any doubts that humans have been experimenting with positions and their bodies since ancient times.

While some have hypothesized that these murals and art functioned as a "menu" for paying clientele, it is far more likely that the erotic pieces were simply intended to arouse the viewer (perhaps giving them some ideas to try), on par with how pornography is used today. Of all the stimuli that can lead to arousal, perceiving the act of sex is the one shared across all cultures. Seeing, or sometimes hearing, sex leads to a natural arousal. It is no wonder, then, that even since ancient times, humans have worked out a way to profit from these biological reactions—images of sex guarantee the increased arousal of the clientele and perhaps upsell them extra services.

This helps us understand the depictions of phalluses spread throughout the city. Some have speculated that they were advertising, pointing the way to the nearest brothel. But it is far more likely that these phalluses were in fact powerful symbols, functioning as an emblem of good fortune and protection that could ward off ill-intending visitors and the evil eye. Archaeologists have found phallic emblems in amulets, as part of frescoes, displayed as statues, and even formed into lamps. These phalluses were referred to as *fascinus* and, according to the Roman author Pliny, were carried by babies and soldiers alike to provide protection. To steal an iconic line from *Buffy the Vampire Slayer*, "Nothing can defeat the penis!"

In the same way as we can be molded by the material we consume, this material can be shaped by events in our cultural landscape. Nothing has made this quite so apparent as our recent experience of the COVID-19 pandemic. The pandemic had a clear impact on our pornographic interests, as shown by the top searches on Pornhub in 2021 in comparison to 2019* (which isn't much different from lists in the preceding years).

---

* Pornhub's insights for 2020 have not, for whatever reason, been made available to the public.

2019

1.	Japanese	**6.**	Asian
2.	Hentai	**7.**	Step Mom
3.	Lesbian	**8.**	Massage
4.	MILF	**9.**	Anal
5.	Korean	**10.**	Ebony

This series of searches is quite notably dominated by fetish interests. "Massage" and "anal" are the only practical descriptors on this list. Now, let's compare this to 2021:

2021

1.	Hentai	**6.**	Challenge
2.	Romance	**7.**	Transgender
3.	Group Sex	**8.**	Goth
4.	Fitness	**9.**	Roommate
5.	Swapping	**10.**	How To . . .

Hentai is the only search to have survived the pandemic (as we shall soon see, penis-shaped krakens are notoriously hard to kill). This list is dominated by genres involving multiple human bodies, such as romance, group sex, swapping, and roommate. The influence that periods of lockdown would have had on each of these fantasies is understandable. While "romance" is a common category on porn sites (though rarely listed in top searches), this search more than doubled in 2021. As Dr. Laurie Betito has remarked, "Human connection has become far more important this past pandemic year. Many people have experienced loneliness and isolation and may be craving love, intimacy and romance. So the next best thing to a partner, it seems, are the fantasies of romance."

Similarly, it's easy to see the appeal of group sex and swapping* (or literally any activity involving a group) after long periods of restriction surrounding how many people we could have contact with. This fantasy may not have been limited to couples longing for a little more spice in their isolation. Lockdown brought obvious limitations of our sexual possibilities. I imagine I'm far from alone in hearing a number of stories of hookups that took, or almost took, place between housemates and friends throughout this time. (The increase in "roommate" fantasies is almost certainly related to this.) For many people, the introduction of bubble buddies or bubble households† meant thinking in terms of sexual interest rather than social interaction. Especially for many single people, selecting which household to "bubble" with could come with considerations of forming a friendship with benefits, trialing a new romantic possibility, or even joining a romantic partnership that was already established. I would not be surprised if questions surrounding "group sex" experimentation were also found under the "how to" search category.

With the dominance of home workouts and YouTube fitness regimes, it is easy to see how "fitness" also slipped into our fantasies. It takes only a few clicks to veer away from a ten-minute abs workout to another video that will work up a similar sweat without your stomach muscles aching the next day.

YouTube wasn't the only social media app that influenced the world of porn. I feel confident in stating that the growth of TikTok was behind the unprecedented rise of "challenge" as a popular porn search term, as well as increased interest in the goth aesthetic, which has been repopularized by Gen Z. In fact, many of these challenges *replicated* popular trends that were going around TikTok, such as the "no nut November" challenge and the "buss-it" challenge (a costume-transformation trend to Erica Banks's song "Buss It"). These videos were sexualized interpretations of trends on

---

* A term that here refers to the swapping of sexual or romantic partners. This encompasses the concept of "swinging" couples, established partners who engage in sexual relationships with other people's partners as well.

† For those not familiar with the term, many cities introduced the concept of "bubbling" with another household during periods of lockdown. This was generally designed for (though not entirely limited to) people living alone. To counter the negative effects of complete social isolation, another household could be nominated to create a "social bubble" with your own.

these apps, or sexualized stories made up about people trying this trend ("Banned from TikTok! Buss-it challenge but he accidentally came inside me" is the name of an actual video on the website). This crept into our fantasies.

The 2021 statistics capture how much our fantasies are directly influenced by the external world. The pandemic affected us all differently, but it did affect nearly everyone. And this is reflected, out of the billions of views that Pornhub received, in our searches.

Our fantasies are a way to escape reality. However, one of the paradoxical features of any good escapist fantasy is its rooting in a somewhat relatable reality. This likely explains why, even in our desperation to forget the pandemic for at least a minute a day, "quarantine" led the search on Pornhub, along with many other similar sites, in 2020. For the majority of us, this was the first time we had experienced anything like these periods of isolation. In many ways, our fantasies felt more real than reality. In these times, we can turn to fictional realities—like pornography—to make sense of what is going on in our lived experience.

Early in 2020, I remember seeing a screenshot of a porn film going viral across media outlets. This was before the impacts of the pandemic were truly felt here in Australia. The film was of two people in a lockdown facility in Wuhan who decided to "find comfort" with each other despite their masks and gloves. To a somewhat COVID-free country, this video seemed bizarre. I thought at the time that it was weirdly sweet. Just like work, family, and friendships, we had to learn how love and relationships would function in this brave new world. Pornography began to depict the shifts long before many other forms of media. It's no wonder that views rose so drastically, if this was the one world holding a mirror (and inspiration) up to our immediate, uncanny experience.

All that being said, there's still one question to answer: How the hell does hentai fit into all this? If you've scoured the internet long enough, it's likely you've come across the term. *Hentai seiyoku* translates in English as "perverse sexual desire," defined by the *Oxford English Dictionary*—it was added in 2011—as a subgenre of Japanese manga and anime with overtly sexualized characters and sexually explicit images and plots. You may have scrolled past hentai before without even realizing it (or you may have been *very* aware of it). This category of pornography is no small player in the game. In 2019, Pornhub reported that it was the second most popular search term on their website—a truly sizable achievement considering there were forty-two billion visits to the site that year. The interest in hentai has only continued to grow. By 2021, it became the number one search term globally on Pornhub, overtaking "Japanese" and even the USA's number one search for "lesbian."

While hentai can consist of cartoon humans performing typically human acts, one of the primary appeals is that it opens the realm of the erotic into the weird, wacky, and whimsical. Hentai is limited only by the boundaries of human creativity and imagination. While it would be an impossible task to summarize all the fantastical inclusions, some of the more popular tropes include: graphically oversize body parts, characters with animal-like characteristics, forced alien pregnancies, seduction by sexy succulent plants—and, perhaps most curiously to many people, a shitload of tentacles.

Tentacle pornography originated in the Edo period of Japan, with a series of woodblock prints depicting women being assaulted by octopuses. One of the earliest ex-

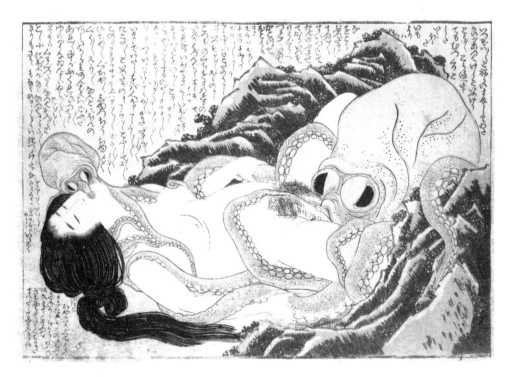

The Dream of the Fisherman's Wife by Hokusai

amples, which remains a popular artwork today, is *The Dream of the Fisherman's Wife* by Hokusai (the artist who famously painted *The Wave*) in 1814. The print depicts two octopuses and one woman. The larger octopus is dexterously performing cunnilingus on the woman, while the smaller octopus (a true multitasker) passionately kisses the woman while playing with her left nipple.

Images such as Hokusai's reference the popular fable of Princess Tamatori, a shell diver who vows to find a pearl stolen from her husband's family by the god of the sea, Ryūjin. Diving to the undersea palace, Tamatori soon finds herself pursued by the sea god's merciless army. Caring more about her sworn vow than her own well-being, she cuts her breast open to hide the jewel inside and makes her way back to the surface. Ultimately, Tamatori is successful in her promise, but dies soon after her escape from the wound that she gave herself. Pearl, 1. Wife, 0.

Hokusai's painting is not only a reference to this fable, but a positive adaptation for its rather grim ending. Instead of performing self-mutilation and then dying, Princess Tamatori is here punished only by the sweet, sweet tongues of two *inkredible* lovers. James Heaton and Toyoshima Mizuho have translated the text that surrounds the image thus.

LARGE OCTOPUS: My wish comes true at last, this day of days; finally I have you in my grasp! Your "bobo" is ripe and full, how wonderful! Superior to all others! To suck and suck and suck some more. After we do it masterfully, I'll guide you to the Dragon Palace of the Sea God and envelop you. Zuu sufu sufu chyu chyu chyu tsu zuu fufufuuu . . .

MAIDEN: You hateful octopus! Your sucking at the mouth of my womb makes me gasp for breath! Aah! yes . . . it's . . . there!!! With the sucker, the sucker!! Inside, squiggle, squiggle, oooh! Oooh, good, oooh good! There, there! Theeeeere! Goood! Whew! Aah! Good, good, aaaaaaaaaah! Not yet! Until now it was I that men called an octopus! An octopus! Ooh! Whew! How are you able . . . !? Ooh! yoyoyooh, saa . . . hicha hicha gucha gucha, yuchyuu chyu guzu guzu suu suuu.

The story—which once ended in the princess's death, and then was reimagined to include her sexual assault—is now recast as a mutually beneficial experience, with octopus and princess alike getting as much as they are giving. A sort of *squid pro quo*, if you will.

How has tentacle erotica continued to pique interest today? Well, I had an *inkling* that there was more to the story. Increased censorship of pornography begins in Japan during the Meiji period, particularly in response to the imposition of Western thought and culture during the war. Artists could face serious consequences if they painted sexual scenes or even naked genitalia. Luckily, they had a solution at hand (all eight of them, in fact). Tentacle erotica provided the perfect substitute for penile objects, and octopuses' handy hands were perfect for covering up anything that shouldn't be seen. Did sex with an aquatic creature even classify as sex? This was a loophole that many artists could use to their advantage. As discussed in an interview with the prolific manga artist Toshio Maeda:

> *It was illegal to create a sensual scene in bed. I thought I should do something to avoid drawing such a normal sensual scene. So I just created a creature. [His tentacle] is not a [penis] as a pretext. I could say, as an excuse, this is not a penis; this is just a part of the creature. You know, the creatures, they don't have a gender. A creature is a creature. So it is not obscene—not illegal.*

There are many examples of things becoming eroticized or fetishized due to constant cultural exposure—I think it's fair to say tentacle erotica has become one of those things. It has become such a common sexual fantasy it even features in Netflix's hit show *Sex Education*. In season two (released in 2020), the fictional high school puts on the only version of *Romeo and Juliet* I will now watch—an intergalactic alien orgy filled with penises and vaginas. Dancing tentacles with penises fill the stage. This artistic masterpiece has been created from the mind of a student called Lily, who has been exploring her sexuality through alien fantasies. Lily speaks about how she has never found these fantasies—which often incorporate tentacle penetration—to be "dirty" or "bad."

Hentai's sharp rise in popularity and representation in mainstream media over recent years has brought it under the scrutiny of academics, particularly those interested in the question of ethics and influence when it comes to the consumption of pornography. Along with the otherworldly illustrations of many of the featured characters, a part of the hentai universe revolves around themes of violence and molestation. The anime and manga stylings of this media also make it far easier to blur the boundaries when it comes to depictions of age. Considerable debate has surrounded *lolicon*, a subgenre that depicts characters (mainly girls) with childlike characteristics in erotic scenarios. Lolicon is a portmanteau of "Lolita complex," a phrase that came about following the publication of Vladimir Nabokov's controversial novel, *Lolita* (1955). The book centers on the obsession that a middle-aged professor develops for a twelve-year-old girl. With all this in mind, it's easy to see why lolicon pornography may have become a point of concern following its initial boom in the 1980s.

After hearing these facts, many of us would be inclined to condemn hentai creators as having questionable ethics at best and promoting outright dangerous ideology at worst. One side of the argument believes there may be an ethical value to hentai for the very reasons we may be inclined to condemn it: this kind of pornography does not involve the use of real human bodies. Viewers can watch their more extreme fantasies played out without concern for the well-being of the performer(s), with far more assurance of the safety of those involved (both on-set and off-) than can often be provided by producers of live-action porn. The world of fantasy provides a vitally important separation from the real. Some believe that societal ethics cannot travel into this world because this world, in many ways, does not belong to humans. This was a vital point for researchers to establish when it came to lolicon—how separate were these childlike characters from their recognizable real-world references?

Scholars have generally determined that these manga and anime characters have, in fact, taken on a reality of their own. As writer Patrick W. Galbraith has observed:

> *Characters are not compensating for something more "real," but rather are in their fiction the object of affection. This has been described as "finding sexual objects in fiction in itself," which in discussions of lolicon is made explicitly distinct from desire for and abuse of children.*

More than objectified objects, these stylized characters have actually been considered primarily as an expression of "aspects of their creators' or consumers' own identities" that they may not be able to tap into outside a fantastical world. This explanation seems similar to that explored by Lily in *Sex Education*, who explains that the tentacle-filled alien world is a portrayal of sexuality that feels like the most authentic expression of herself. This pornography becomes a sort of paradox, existing within our world while simultaneously being removed from it. Because of this distance, many people are able to find erotic enjoyment that may not be possible if these scenarios were observed in the "real" world—whether because the viewer would be overcome with feelings of empathy that would override their pleasure, or because they would experience shame as a dual result of this pleasure. As described in an essay fittingly titled "Way Better Than Real":

> *The distance of manga and tentacle hentai from the "real" mitigate[s] the most shameful responses—encouraging both rapt engrossment in the fantasy and cold distance from acts of violence, domination, molestation, rape, bondage and torture. . . . The moral distance affected by tentacle hentai and manga also fosters an emotional distancing. Because this genre is cartoon, it prevents reflexive empathy with, or sympathy for, the horrid violation.*

This perspective simultaneously eases and enhances concerns surrounding this specific medium. It gives assurance that the stimulus of arousal—specifically one that is rooted in violence—has no substitute or basis in the "real" world. However, for this to be the case, this state of eroticism must necessarily also be removed from empathetic, emotional feeling. This opens a whole new can of sea worms. Should we consume pornography that is removed from feelings of human sympathy? What are the dangers, if any, of doing so? And what are the benefits of seeking out pornography that is grounded in practices of empathy and connectivity?

The Power of Pornography

History teaches us that the power of pornography is more than just skin-deep. It has the ability to affect and alter our behaviors, emotions, and opinions. If, as we have seen, the impact of this susceptibility surpasses the walls of the bedroom, then it is vital that we become more conscious consumers. One easy way for us to do that is by engaging with "ethical pornography," a phrase I did not hear until far too long into my own viewership.

Many of us have been guilty of watching pornography without much thought of where it came from. Even if the thought has occurred to you, the shooting conditions of "bIg titted blonde gets f#Cked by NOT-brother" can be pretty hard to research. As we place increasing emphasis on being conscious consumers in all other aspects of our lives, such as considering the environmental impact of the food we consume or the production environments of the clothes we purchase, why doesn't this same logic apply to pornography?

I think it's because of the taboo; it's easy to sustain cognitive dissonance between the video in front of us and the conditions under which it was produced. The exploitation and systemic disregard of sex workers' rights are gradually gaining wider awareness, though we still have a long way to go. The ways in which we unknowingly contribute to it, however, are rarely discussed. If we're ever to normalize the consumption of pornography, it's imperative that we start subjecting it to the same moral principles applied elsewhere, and making the switch to ethical pornography is one practical solution.

Broadly defined, pornography is deemed ethical if it is made legally, respects the rights of the workers, provides safe and good working conditions, produces both fantasy and real-world sex, and celebrates diversity among performers. There is an abundance of sites that now support, host, and create ethical pornographic media. Unlike on the sets for many erotic films found on more mainstream sites, the producers of these films ensure all performers have personal boundaries and limits respected, have given explicit consent for every act performed, have the right to stop shooting the moment they feel uncomfortable, and receive basic labor rights and fair pay.

It is not just performers and creatives who benefit from the consumption of ethical pornography: watching these videos can provide unexpected advantages for the consumer. This was an aspect that I didn't anticipate when I made the switch to these websites, and it changed my relationship to contemporary pornography. There was an enhanced sense of sexual satisfaction to be gained from watching performers who I could trust were comfortable with what they were doing. The increased care given to the production quality equally offered a more intimate and intense sense of immersion in the scenes, which differed greatly from any experience with digital porn that I'd had before. These videos were able to tap into a sense of empathy and compassion, words that I'd rarely connected with the pornography industry.

This can have real-world effects. Watching porn that prioritizes the sexual satisfaction of all parties could logically encourage us to do so within our own sex lives. More than this, many of these videos provide models for how to introduce fantasy play into our sex practices. I find this particularly true of ethical porn films that venture into the world of BDSM. It is common for this genre of production to include a conversation at the start between the participants, in which they discuss their desires, limits, and safe words. This is a small inclusion but a critical one. It establishes a separation between the real world and "play," providing instruction on how these can be clearly and safely switched between. This, in turn, legitimizes the wide range of desires that live under this umbrella.

Opening a pornographic film with this behind-the-scenes-style discussion shows that this conversation isn't just the boring admin before the fun begins—it helps to makes communication sexy. Hearing people talk openly and honestly about their sexual desires is shown to be an enthralling experience. It creates a fiery anticipation about the forthcoming play and allows the participants to feel empowered and in control as they step into the fantasy situation. The result for the viewer is what appears to be genuine sexual satisfaction and fulfillment playing from their smartphone, which guarantees to never set off their BS detector.

Ethical porn can provide far more than momentary sexual enjoyment, and it's worth any monetary cost. In my experience with capitalism, "free" and "ethical" are rarely complementary ideals—someone is paying the price for it somewhere. If you have the means to make this investment, it's orgasmic in itself that for nine dollars a month, I can switch my vibrator to high and go to town guilt-free, knowing my money's going toward creating better conditions for sex workers and toward paying creatives. As awareness increases and ethical pornography sites rise, more of the sites *do* offer viewers access for free, with the trade-off of watching advertisements before the video begins. Whatever our situations, there are small changes we can make to more ethically consume pornography.

Let's take a turn from the production of porn to looking at the many ways we consume it. Why do we watch pornography in the first place? This is a human phenomenon. No other animals keep sexy snaps of each other hidden under their beds in case they're struggling to get in the mood, but engaging with pornography is a behavior shared by an increasing majority of the human population. In 2014, the Australian national survey reported that 63 percent of men and 20 percent of women had looked at pornography in the previous year. By 2016, it was reported that five in six men (84 percent), and one in two women (54 percent) admitted to watching pornographic media. By 2022, our survey gathered data on who had purposely watched sex on the internet as follows:

CIS WOMEN: 73.5 percent

CIS MEN: 88.3 percent

NONBINARY/NONCONFORMING: 77.1 percent

TRANS WOMEN: 80.2 percent

TRANS MEN: 78.1 percent

OTHER: 80.9 percent

Similar increases are being reported all over the world. A report from Poland stated that the "estimated number of general population members viewing pornography on the Internet increased over three times (310%) between October 2004 and October 2016—starting from an estimated 2.76 million in the first period to 8.54 million in the last." While in 2004, 8 percent of the population was watching internet porn, this had tripled to 24 percent by 2016—a fact that could also be explained by greater access to the internet.

So why exactly do we—as a rational, intelligent, (allegedly) evolved species—do it? The primary reason that people report is simply because it increases their sex drive. It adds further sensory elements to masturbatory practices, excites the imagination, and can help to quicken orgasms. (A shout-out to respondents who reported they watched porn "for the story and the script.") Less commonly, though still prominently, porn is reported as a way to enhance sexual performance. Who said you can't teach an old dog new tricks? Answers that fall under this category—such as teaching new positions, improved understanding of pleasure experiences of the opposite sex, and even as a form of sex education—account for nearly 10 percent of the reasons people watch porn.

This reason for turning to porn is ostensibly on the rise. "How to" searches on Pornhub rose in 2021 by 245 percent, making this category the tenth most popular across the site. Most popular among these searches were ones that would fall under sex education: how to put on a condom, how to finger yourself, how to shave balls, and how to find the G-spot. These queries—like how to put on a condom—reveal the fact that these sites are beginning to be used as a horned-up search engine as well as for the consumption of pornography. It may be the case that because these sites aren't heavily censored, users feel they receive more informative and instructional information there than they would from a wikiHow guide.

I can vouch for the difference in educational quality. When my first boyfriend started throwing terms like *hand job* and *blow job* out there, I could not have been more clueless, and so I ended up on the most bizarre wikiHow tutorial I have ever seen. I was even more confused than when I started . . . until Google took me to porn-site tutorials (thanks, bestie). These videos aimed to educate rather than arouse. They walked through everything from basic instructions to more skillful techniques, and how to communicate with your partner about your wants and needs. This sexy encyclopedia became an invaluable tool as I began my sexual exploration. It gave me an understanding of the range of sexual activities, as well as an idea of what I did and did not want to try.

Of course, our motives for watching other people get down with their bad selves from the comfort of our iPhones don't always have to be productive. Following increased sex drive and sexual performance, social reasons are quoted to be the next largest category for pornography use. This includes things such as "because all of my friends are watching it" and "for the quality of the actors," along with more aesthetic reasons, such as "I paint nudes and it is my source of inspiration" and simply "for entertainment." Because giant pornography sites such as Pornhub and Redtube dominate our cultural perception of pornography, we tend to forget that erotic media can also be an artform. Just like with our consumption of romantic novels and the Marvel cinematic universe, we don't always need a sexual reason to consume pornography. This is, perhaps, an example of when pornography is an erotic experience rather than a sexual one. It can excite the imagination and body, while not necessarily leading to or inspiring sexual thoughts or behavior. Sometimes porn is just . . . porn.

Considering the sizable debate that envelops "unhealthy" consumption of pornography, the motives that would fall under this category are low. The fourth category of reasons for why we watch porn has been identified by this study as its ability to fill a lack in relationships or emotional skills. This accounted for about 3.8 percent of the total variance. Now, not every motive within this category would be flagged as a point of concern. This includes turning to pornography because of an absence of a romantic partner, because a long time has passed since being sexually active, or because of a need for love. Other reasons—such as turning to pornography to relieve stress or to distract from stressful thoughts—*could* lead to more problematic engagement (though this is far from guaranteed).

When *does* engagement with pornography become problematic, then? If we were to ask a random group of strangers on the street, it's likely they would say it becomes problematic when excessive violence or other "taboo" subjects are depicted. However, problematic engagement seems to be determined in these studies more by motivation rather than by content depicted—in particular, stress-motivated usage seems to be the defining feature. Masturbation, often aided by pornography, can be a class-A way to relieve stress. It releases all those make-happy-now chemicals in your body so you can forget your worries, if only for a couple of minutes, and simply experience bodily pleasure. This isn't an issue in itself—this motivation becomes an issue only when it becomes a *compulsive* means to relieve stress, which is ubiquitous in our busy lives. Even more so than other stress-relieving methods that can develop into addictions, such as alcohol or weed (in places where consumption is legal), pornography is an "easily accessible, affordable, seemingly anonymous and fast way to diminish stress." But turning to this as constant stress relief can, paradoxically, result in development of even more stress, as pornography becomes a crutch.

An example of this is seen in Netflix's comedy-drama *Bonding* (2018–21). In season two, Tiff, a dominatrix and graduate student living in New York, discusses with her best friend why she masturbates while watching porn. For just a second, she says, it allows her to "zombie out." Later in the episode, after a fight with her friend, Tiff desperately tries to arouse herself on the couch, porn playing on her phone and fingers down her pants. But she is upset from the fight and no amount of "Did someone here order a large pepperoni pizza?" is going to do the trick this time. While this isn't necessarily a case of addiction to pornography, it is an example of when this media is turned to for reasons that *may* become a problem—that is, to relieve stress and distract from troubling thoughts. Tiff wasn't in the mood for sex—she was feeling anything but sexy. She wasn't motivated to turn to porn for any reason other than the promise of "zombieing out" for a second. If that kind of dependence goes unchecked, it *could* become a problem.

While overconsumption of pornography is often discussed and debated as a wide-ranging concern, the number of people who suffer from porn addiction is low. In the Second Australian Study of Health and Relationships it accounted for around 4 percent of men and 1 percent of women who participated. Pornography users also generally reported high levels of positive effects in comparison to the negatives. Fifty-eight percent of respondents thought pornography had had a very positive or a positive effect on their attitudes toward sexuality (35 percent felt it had had no effect and 7 percent thought it had a negative effect or a large negative effect). These effects included:

> *feeling less repressed about sex; feeling more open-minded about sex; increased tolerance of other people's sexualities; giving pleasure to consumers; providing educational insights; sustaining sexual interest in long-term relationships; making consumers more attentive to a partner's sexual desires; helping consumers find an identity or community; and helping them to talk to their partners about sex.*

The benefits didn't stop here: 89.9 percent of men and 79.4 percent of women said it enhanced the pleasure of masturbation, and 65.6 percent of men and 53.7 percent of women said it could improve sexual relations among adults. In contrast, only 12.9 percent of men and 10.2 percent of women thought using porn had had a bad effect on them. If so many people are reporting these positives, then why is there such a huge public debate surrounding the industry?

Most of us don't realize quite how big the industry of pornography has become. In 2006, it had larger revenues than Microsoft, Google, Amazon, eBay, Yahoo, Apple, and Netflix *combined*. Its influence has shown no sign of slowing down.

> *The biggest and perhaps best source of data about what people like to watch on the internet and what they would pay for doesn't come from streaming giants like Netflix, Amazon Prime Video, or Hulu. It comes from porn. . . . The porn industry could have a bigger economic influence on the US than Netflix. Revenue estimates are as high as $97 billion (Netflix brings in about $11.7 billion).*

With this kind of hold on society, it is absolutely vital that we know and discuss its impact and influence, both for those involved in production and for us as consumers. Pornography, and earlier forms of erotic art, has had a significant impact throughout human history. It has told the story of our gods, it has critiqued our political authorities, and it has brought about revolution. The size of the industry today—and the monopoly that a few giant corporations have on the landscape—means its power over us may be greater than ever before. We must be aware of who holds this power and what they are using it for. In this way, we can take the power back when it comes to sexual media, and find ways in which it can ethically benefit our well-being and be a productive part of sexuality for those of us who want it.

The final plates are being cleared. The last droplets of the wine are being poured, and the general chatter is beginning to subside. Victor Hugo has fallen asleep at the table, Joyce's cat has found its way into his lap. Guests are attending to their last-minute business (John Wilmot is placing a considerably large order from Mrs. Phillips's shop). In high spirits, we begin to pick ourselves up from the table, gathering all the books and illustrations that have been left about. We can return them to the library on our way out.

AFTERCARE

It may well be asked why, at a time like this, I think sex is an important subject for conversation—why, while our news stations report daily on the effects of our heating planet, acts of inconceivable cruelty, and other "unprecedented" events, I think public discourse needs to involve more dildos, strap-ons, and cock rings. I don't ask us to talk about sex as a distraction from these troubled times. Weirdly enough, I believe that talking about it will provide at least part of a solution for those troubles.

Empathy is at the heart of sex and sexuality—or it should be. When we look back through history into the proclivities of those who came before us, and we take these stories and see what they can teach us about our world today, we are using empathy. So many of the troubles that currently plague our world are the result of disconnection from the earth, each other, and ourselves.

Sex is the antithesis of disconnection. It can engender a deeply intimate relationship with your own body or the body of another human. It can ground us, it can produce life, it can make us feel alive. Every single person, in one form or another, has a relationship with sex and sexuality. It can be considered our driving force, a sacred act, or simply no more than the act that probably brought us into the world and one we want no further relationship with. In some way or another, all our lives are touched by sex. That is a fact that no one is able to escape. So why would we not want that relationship to be rooted in empowerment and empathy?

For far too long, sexuality has been used against us, though this wasn't always the case. For many, many years, humans enjoyed sex lives that were relatively free of stigma and shame—concepts nearly all of us have had to encounter in our modern sexual journeys. Demonizing an act essential to human survival has perhaps been one of the most successful efforts of mass policing. As we look back to cultural shifts in history—the criminalization of homosexuality, the prosecution of "licentious" women, the war on masturbation—we see a clear pattern emerging. The vilification of our sensual enjoyment has less to do with a genuine concern surrounding sex and more to do with the expectation of positive political or social outcomes for the vilifier.

In talking about sex, we do not merely "take the power back"—we are called upon to remember that this power was always ours to begin with. By painting the diversity of our sexual experiences back into history, we create a foundation for better practices today—taking us to that all-important place of empowerment and empathy.

These are big expectations for one book to achieve. However, when you close this book and return it to its shelf, the conversation is far from over. This book is not an end point; it is a conversation starter. I hope you've found at least one story that resonated with you, something that made you laugh out loud, a fact that disrupted your own understanding, and ideas that inspire many wonderful conversations of your own.

When I began my journey of digging up the horny secrets of history, it was a sense of community and connection that inspired me. It was the way people would come together to laugh at a peculiar object from the past, or the collective shock at a fact that disrupts presumptions about a period. Most especially, it was the moment when someone saw a tidbit from history and said to themselves, "They were just like me." These are the moments that make this work worth doing. This is why I think it is so important. Sex brings people together. It is an abundant source of connection—one that, paradoxically, isn't always strictly sexual. It can be humorous and playful, inquisitive and conversational.

Sex generates life in more ways than one, and we can harness that power to create something truly wonderful.

Instead of trying to iron out our kinks, it's time we embraced them. It's time we took all the paradoxical and contradictory parts of our sexual history and used them as reference points to guide us forward. Perhaps we will not solve all the world's issues in one sitting. Real change takes time, and the first trickles often look insignificant. But these small changes build up—these choices we make to treat ourselves with more kindness, to see others with more accepting eyes. Our journey toward climax can take some time, but each act of foreplay will gradually move us there. Until one day, BOOM! We may be left with an orgasmic explosion of empathy and understanding.

For now, it is time to grab our coats and hats. Say farewell to the friends you have met tonight and give your calling card to those you would like to see again. There goes Aristotle, supporting Augustine on his shoulder. There is Sappho, making friends with Stein and Woolf. Out go Katharine Davis and Alfred Kinsey, Krafft-Ebing and Aristophanes. Let's thank them all for the wonderful and dynamic conversation they led for us tonight.

As we watch them all leave—with whips in hands and pens composing ballads to the glory of the dildo—let us remember this is not the end, but just a beginning. This is your formal invitation to host a dinner party of your very own. Take all you have learned tonight, and all you have ever known, and place it in a dynamic, wide-ranging conversation.

Our history is as full of kinks as our path toward the future will be, filled with twists and turns and exceptions to the rules. That is how all good history happens—history that you will help us write.

Leave this place carrying with you the same comfort and warmth you met inside. Remember, you are always welcome here. Whenever you want to return, you will be greeted. Victor Hugo will be dancing in the library, Gertrude Stein will be lecturing around the dining table. Hans Christian Andersen will be writing secretly in his diary, and Sigmund Freud will still be pulling out his hair about the enigma of femininity. We will all be here, with open arms, waiting for you to join us again in discussion.

But for now, in the eloquent words of Wolfgang Mozart:

I wish you a good night.
Shit in the bed with all your might.
Sleep with peace on your mind.
And try to kiss your own behind.

Embrace your existence in this chaotically beautiful kinky history we share—and I hope you continue talking about sex.

Acknowledgments

I would like to dedicate this book to the important teachers I've had in my own life.

To my friends, who have continually taught me selflessness.

To my partner, who taught me what it really means to believe in yourself.

To my grandparents, who taught me the strength of resilience.

To my dad, who first taught me the power of stories and the magic of words.

To my mum, who told me that this magic is real—and it lives in every act of kindness and bravery.

And to my most significant teacher, my brother, Ewan. Thank you for reminding me that love will always burn brighter than any flames of hatred.

You are the reason we will be able to make history.

We would also like to extend our thanks to the incredible supports who made this book possible. To Pantera Press—especially Tom Langshaw, who first imagined this book's potential—thank you for always believing in and trusting our vision (even when we weren't sure what it would look like). To the University of Melbourne, which has been an invaluable support to both of us over the past decade. To Mary McGillivray, whose work first helped inspire the idea of *Kinky History*. To Ewan's amazing care team—with special thanks to Sharon McCrory—whose hard work and dedication have made it possible for us to write this book. And finally, to Chris Russell, who was always there ready with a gin and tonic for us at the end of a long day of writing.

Appendix:
SexTistics Survey Details

The SexTistics survey was an anonymous online survey launched in April 2022. The questions were devised so that the wording was comparable to some of the questions asked in national studies such as the Australian Study of Health and Relationships. In less than a fortnight the survey had already received over ten thousand responses. The link for the survey was disseminated through social media via TikTok, Instagram, and Facebook. As the respondents were largely existing followers of the Kinky History and/or the SexTistics series, there will be some inherent biases and, therefore, we do not claim that these results are reflective of the general population. However, as there were a total of 14,058 completed responses, the sample size means this is not a survey to be ignored.

This appendix does not comprise an analysis or a full report of the data; the following pages merely contain a small snapshot of some of key demographics and statistics that have been quoted in this book.

When considering this data, it should be borne in mind that the surveys were conducted at the beginning of 2022. Many questions referred to the participants' behaviors over the previous twelve months, which may well have been affected by changes in environmental factors due to COVID-19 and the subsequent restrictions and lockdowns.

We would like to thank all the respondents who took the time to participate in our survey.

Table 1: Demographic characteristics of participants

	FEMALE		MALE		NONBINARY	
	N	%	N	%	N	%
Gender identity	9485	67.47%	2891	20.56%	1089	7.75%
Primary residence						
United States of America	5808	41.60%	1794	12.85%	654	4.68%
Australia	858	6.14%	274	1.96%	89	0.64%
United Kingdom	704	5.04%	233	1.67%	76	0.54%
Canada	473	3.39%	126	0.90%	41	0.29%
Other	1582	11.33%	445	3.19%	220	1.58%
Age group						
16–19	1760	12.52%	493	3.51%	396	2.82%
20–29	4526	32.20%	982	6.99%	518	3.68%
30–39	2280	16.22%	708	5.04%	136	0.97%
40–49	679	4.83%	399	2.84%	22	0.16%
50–59	188	1.34%	207	1.47%	8	0.06%
60–69	19	0.14%	61	0.43%	1	0.01%
70–79	4	0.03%	15	0.11%	1	0.01%
Highest level of education						
Less than high school	104	0.74%	39	0.28%	25	0.18%
High school	3256	23.20%	1073	7.64%	582	4.15%
College certificate or diploma	2311	16.46%	763	5.44%	205	1.46%
Undergraduate university degree	2692	19.18%	695	4.95%	195	1.39%
Postgraduate university degree	1112	7.92%	314	2.24%	80	0.57%

TRANS WOMEN		TRANS MEN		OTHER		NO RESPONSE		OVERALL	
N	%	N	%	N	%	N	%	N	%
81	0.58%	216	1.54%	251	1.79%	45	0.32%	14058	100.00%
137	0.98%	20	0.14%	133	0.95%	47	0.34%	8593	61.54%
25	0.18%	6	0.04%	14	0.10%	6	0.04%	1272	9.11%
17	0.12%	7	0.05%	24	0.17%	13	0.09%	1074	7.69%
10	0.07%		0.00%	14	0.10%	3	0.02%	667	4.78%
57	0.41%	12	0.09%	30	0.21%	11	0.08%	2357	16.88%
32	0.23%	122	0.87%	120	0.85%	26	0.18%	2949	20.98%
22	0.16%	80	0.57%	95	0.68%	15	0.11%	6238	44.37%
19	0.14%	10	0.07%	26	0.18%	3	0.02%	3182	22.63%
5	0.04%	3	0.02%	7	0.05%		0.00%	1115	7.93%
2	0.01%	1	0.01%	1	0.01%	1	0.01%	408	2.90%
1	0.01%		0.00%		0.00%		0.00%	82	0.58%
	0.00%		0.00%		0.00%		0.00%	20	0.14%
1	0.01%	12	0.09%	6	0.04%	3	0.02%	190	1.35%
48	0.34%	132	0.94%	149	1.06%	31	0.22%	5271	37.55%
15	0.11%	33	0.24%	34	0.24%	8	0.06%	3369	24.00%
15	0.11%	32	0.23%	45	0.32%	1	0.01%	3675	26.18%
1	0.01%	7	0.05%	15	0.11%	2	0.01%	1531	10.91%

Table 2: Sexual identity, attraction, and experience by gender

	FEMALE		MALE		NONBINARY	
	N	%	N	%	N	%
Gender identity	9485	67.47%	2891	20.56%	1089	7.75%
Sexual identity						
Heterosexual	3717	39.19%	1765	61.05%	14	1.29%
Bisexual	3689	38.89%	515	17.81%	347	31.86%
Homosexual	308	3.25%	369	12.76%	148	13.59%
Asexual	202	2.13%	25	0.86%	82	7.53%
Queer	452	4.77%	54	1.87%	270	24.79%
Other	633	6.67%	97	3.36%	197	18.09%
Undecided	484	5.10%	66	2.28%	31	2.85%
Sexual attraction						
Exclusively female	141	1.49%	1311	45.35%	87	7.99%
Predominantly female	757	7.98%	909	31.44%	277	25.44%
Equally	2606	27.47%	164	5.67%	424	38.93%
Predominantly male	4289	45.22%	265	9.17%	179	16.44%
Exclusively male	1510	15.92%	226	7.82%	31	2.85%
No one	179	1.89%	12	0.42%	88	8.08%
No response	3	0.03%	4	0.14%	3	0.28%
Sexual experience						
Exclusively female	204	2.15%	1489	51.50%	132	12.12%
Predominantly female	237	2.50%	578	19.99%	123	11.29%
Equally	489	5.16%	81	2.80%	139	12.76%
Predominantly male	2981	31.43%	148	5.12%	286	26.26%
Exclusively male	4666	49.19%	311	10.76%	215	19.74%
No one	899	9.48%	277	9.58%	192	17.63%
No response	9	0.09%	7	0.24%	2	0.18%

TRANS WOMEN		TRANS MEN		OTHER		NO RESPONSE		OVERALL	
N	%	N	%	N	%	N	%	N	%
81	0.58%	216	1.54%	251	1.79%	45	0.32%	14058	100.00%
4	4.94%	10	4.63%	12	4.78%	1	2.22%	5523	39.29%
35	43.21%	80	37.04%	69	27.49%	11	24.44%	4746	33.76%
13	16.05%	30	13.89%	26	10.36%	6	13.33%	900	6.40%
1	1.23%	11	5.09%	12	4.78%	4	8.89%	337	2.40%
14	17.28%	39	18.06%	31	12.35%	6	13.33%	866	6.16%
9	11.11%	37	17.13%	96	38.25%	11	24.44%	1080	7.68%
5	6.17%	9	4.17%	5	1.99%	6	13.33%	606	4.31%
8	9.88%	9	4.17%	22	8.76%	5	11.11%	1583	11.26%
32	39.51%	42	19.44%	46	18.33%	10	22.22%	2073	14.75%
23	28.40%	70	32.41%	104	41.43%	16	35.56%	3407	24.24%
15	18.52%	66	30.56%	41	16.33%	7	15.56%	4862	34.59%
1	1.23%	16	7.41%	15	5.98%	2	4.44%	1801	12.81%
2	2.47%	13	6.02%	21	8.37%	5	11.11%	320	2.28%
	0.00%		0.00%	2	0.80%		0.00%	12	0.09%
18	22.22%	35	16.20%	29	11.55%	5	11.11%	1912	13.60%
14	17.28%	23	10.65%	22	8.76%	3	6.67%	1000	7.11%
11	13.58%	32	14.81%	29	11.55%	3	6.67%	784	5.58%
14	17.28%	40	18.52%	47	18.73%	7	15.56%	3523	25.06%
9	11.11%	41	18.98%	65	25.90%	13	28.89%	5320	37.84%
15	18.52%	45	20.83%	57	22.71%	14	31.11%	1499	10.66%
	0.00%		0.00%	2	0.80%		0.00%	20	0.14%

Table 3: Percentages of respondents who thought the following counted as sex

	FEMALE	MALE	NON-BINARY	TRANS WOMEN	TRANS MEN	OTHER	NO RESPONSE	OVERALL
Vaginal intercourse	99.69%	99.20%	99.54%	100.00%	99.07%	98.80%	100.00%	99.56%
Anal intercourse	96.76%	96.95%	97.98%	98.77%	97.22%	96.41%	95.56%	96.90%
Oral sex	73.00%	75.11%	85.74%	87.65%	87.96%	80.40%	82.22%	74.90%
Manual stimulation	37.74%	34.54%	54.81%	49.38%	52.58%	45.97%	60.00%	38.92%
Deep kissing	3.05%	5.70%	5.11%	6.17%	4.69%	4.84%	13.33%	3.86%

Table 4: Participation rates for partnered sexual activity

	FEMALE	MALE	NON-BINARY	TRANS WOMEN	TRANS MEN	OTHER	NO RESPONSE	OVERALL
Have ever participated in								
Vaginal intercourse	85.88%	75.79%	70.65%	62.96%	68.84%	65.34%	53.33%	81.76%
Anal intercourse	55.85%	68.28%	47.01%	62.96%	40.93%	37.85%	26.67%	57.12%
Oral sex	87.76%	88.17%	76.54%	79.01%	73.49%	70.52%	57.78%	86.30%
Manual Stimulation	88.18%	87.31%	79.02%	75.31%	77.21%	70.92%	57.78%	86.65%
Mean frequency in past 4 weeks								
Vaginal intercourse	4.8	4.1	3.3	1.2	2.8	3.3	3.7	
Anal intercourse	0.4	1.3	0.5	1.1	0.5	0.4	1.5	
Oral sex	4.6	3.8	2.8	2.5	2.5	3.0	3.1	

Note: Participants who had earlier answered that they had had no sexual experience with anyone were excluded from this question.

Table 5: Participation rates for autoerotic activities during the past 12 months

	FEMALE	MALE	NON-BINARY	TRANS WOMEN	TRANS MEN	OTHER	NO RESPONSE	OVERALL
Masturbated alone	95.64%	99.06%	96.69%	96.30%	94.44%	97.61%	91.11%	96.43%
Had phone sex or called a telephone sex line	23.12%	23.95%	29.22%	33.33%	33.80%	31.08%	22.22%	24.12%
Went to a sex site on the internet on purpose	73.51%	88.26%	77.05%	80.25%	78.14%	80.88%	71.11%	77.05%
Met a sexual partner through a dating site	16.42%	23.34%	20.50%	19.75%	15.81%	17.27%	4.44%	18.14%
Used a sex toy such as a vibrator, dildo or butt plug	77.85%	56.29%	74.15%	79.01%	78.24%	68.53%	48.89%	72.89%
Been involved in role-playing or dressing up	25.57%	24.22%	31.37%	41.98%	33.80%	29.08%	17.78%	26.00%
Been involved in B&D or S&M	36.10%	32.00%	48.94%	42.50%	47.69%	41.43%	27.27%	36.54%
Been involved in group sex	6.40%	11.33%	13.56%	11.11%	7.41%	8.43%	6.67%	8.05%
Used your fingers to stimulate a partner's anus	17.91%	46.85%	22.19%	30.86%	25.58%	21.20%	15.91%	24.43%
Been involved in oral-anal contact or rimming	22.72%	39.71%	22.51%	32.10%	20.83%	22.80%	13.33%	26.18%

Table 6: Sex toy usage in the past 12 months

	NO	YES	UNSURE
Used a sex toy in the past 12 months	26.55%	72.89%	0.56%
Gender identity			
Female	21.85%	77.85%	0.31%
Male	42.70%	56.29%	1.01%
Nonbinary	24.93%	74.15%	0.92%
Trans women	19.75%	79.01%	1.23%
Trans men	21.76%	78.24%	0.00%
Other	28.69%	68.53%	2.79%
Prefer not to respond	46.67%	48.89%	4.44%
Sexual identity			
Heterosexual	31.90%	67.68%	0.42%
Bisexual	19.32%	80.16%	0.53%
Homosexual	28.29%	70.71%	1.00%
Asexual	54.17%	45.54%	0.30%
Queer	20.74%	78.68%	0.58%
Other	19.93%	79.33%	0.74%
Undecided	36.75%	62.09%	1.16%
Highest level of education			
Less than high school	48.15%	49.74%	2.12%
High school	33.28%	65.98%	0.74%
College certificate or diploma	21.84%	77.74%	0.42%
Undergraduate university degree	23.05%	76.46%	0.49%
Postgraduate university degree	19.24%	80.56%	0.20%
Age group			
16–19	46.46%	52.28%	1.26%
20–29	21.67%	77.88%	0.45%
30–39	18.48%	81.23%	0.28%
40–49	21.44%	78.38%	0.18%
50–59	25.31%	74.69%	0.00%
60–69	52.44%	47.56%	0.00%
70–79	61.11%	38.89%	0.00%

Table 7: Frequency of (solo) masturbation for both the past 12 months and the past 4 weeks

	FEMALE	MALE	NON-BINARY	TRANS WOMEN	TRANS MEN	OTHER	NO RESPONSE	OVERALL
Masturbated in the past 12 months								
No	3.79%	0.76%	2.58%	3.70%	3.70%	1.99%	6.67%	3.05%
Yes	95.64%	99.06%	96.69%	96.30%	94.44%	97.61%	91.11%	96.43%
Not Sure	0.57%	0.17%	0.74%	0.00%	1.85%	0.40%	2.22%	0.52%
Masturbated in the past 4 weeks								
Never	9.57%	2.84%	6.89%	7.41%	6.94%	7.57%	8.89%	7.89%
Less than once a week	24.21%	7.47%	17.91%	9.88%	12.50%	15.54%	24.44%	19.86%
1–3 times a week	42.18%	31.62%	38.11%	34.57%	39.35%	36.65%	33.33%	39.48%
4–6 times a week	17.63%	30.23%	23.42%	33.33%	25.46%	25.10%	13.33%	21.00%
Daily	1.45%	5.12%	2.94%	1.23%	6.02%	2.79%	4.44%	2.43%
More than daily	4.96%	22.73%	10.74%	13.58%	9.72%	12.35%	15.56%	9.35%
Mean number of times in the past 4 weeks								
Heterosexual	7.8	20.7	10.9	14.5	24.8	13.0	20.0	12.0
Bisexual	11.1	23.0	14.2	16.6	15.1	14.4	20.6	12.8
Homosexual	9.7	23.4	16.0	12.3	16.5	11.0	17.3	16.7
Asexual	5.7	15.3	8.6	3.0	7.8	6.5	0.5	7.2
Queer	11.2	29.8	14.1	15.6	14.1	17.1	10.0	13.7
Other	11.0	24.9	12.8	13.7	13.7	13.6	9.9	12.9
Undecided	8.8	23.9	15.9	18.6	3.6	14.4	28.5	11.0
Overall mean	9.5	21.8	13.7	15.3	14.5	13.6	15.4	12.6

Table 8: Average number of lifetime sexual partners by gender and sexual identity

	FEMALE		MALE		NONBINARY		TRANS WOMEN	
	Opposite Sex	Same Sex	Opposite Sex	Same Sex	Opposite Sex	Same Sex	Opposite Sex	Same Sex
	12.2	1.5	16.3	9.6	9.4	7.3	22.3	9.2
Heterosexual	12.3	0.6	17.9	0.4	5.8	0.0	6.3	2.0
Bisexual	13.0	2.0	16.5	7.8	8.8	4.7	14.9	14.7
Homosexual	5.3	5.0	4.8	51.8	5.4	22.5	0.9	2.8
Asexual	2.9	0.4	4.1	2.0	3.2	1.0		
Queer	16.1	2.7	16.4	29.8	13.7	7.4	69.2	7.2
Other	11.4	2.1	22.6	4.9	8.1	3.5	6.4	5.5
Undecided	7.9	0.4	15.5	0.5	14.3	5.9	15.0	2.7

	TRANS MEN		OTHER		NO RESPONSE		OVERALL	
	Opposite Sex	Same Sex	Opposite Sex	Same Sex	Opposite Sex	Same Sex	Opposite Sex	Same Sex
	2.8	2.8	7.5	2.9	3.6	1.9	12.7	3.7
Heterosexual	8.6	8.0	8.8	0.3	20.0		14.0	0.6
Bisexual	2.6	1.6	12.1	4.6	2.0	1.0	12.9	2.9
Homosexual	2.0	5.3	1.8	5.4	0.7	2.3	4.8	28.6
Asexual	2.8	2.2	0.3	1.0	5.0	0.0	3.0	0.7
Queer	3.8	1.8	9.3	1.9	4.5	1.0	15.5	5.8
Other	1.4	4.1	4.8	1.7	3.8	3.1	11.0	2.7
Undecided	2.2	1.0	6.0	1.7	3.0	1.3	8.9	0.8

Image Credits

The Sin Kink

The Pleasure Kink

Queer Kinks

The Kink Kink

The Porn Kink

page 204: Illustration from the Book of the Dead © The Trustees of the British Museum

pages 211–212: *Bacchus et Ariane* by Agostino Carracci, uploaded by Act~commonswiki / Wikimedia Commons / public domain; *Hercule et Dejanire* by Agostino Carracci, uploaded by Act~commonswiki / Wikimedia Commons / public domain; *Alcibiade et Glycere* by Agostino Carracci, uploaded by Act~commonswiki / Wikimedia Commons / public domain

page 220: Erotic scene from . . . the Lupanar . . . in Pompeii, sourced from *Pompeii* by Filippo Coarelli (ed.), uploaded by WolfgangRieger / Wikimedia Commons / public domain

page 225: *Tako to Ama* by Katsushika Hokusai, modified and uploaded by Materialscientist / Wikimedia Commons / public domain

Notes

THE SIN KINK

The Invention of Innocence

4. **"All acts of virtue are prescribed":** Thomas Aquinas, "Question 94, Article 3," *Summa Theologica.*

4. certain actions are "intrinsically evil": Peter Vardy, *The Puzzle of Sex* (London: SCM Press, 2009), 75.

5. "turning a generally negative attitude to sex": Vardy, *Puzzle of Sex,* 52.

5. surrendered himself entirely to the powers: Saint Augustine, Bishop of Hippo, *The Confessions of Saint Augustine,* ed. Temple Scott, trans. Edward Pusey (New York: Stokes, 1910), 33.

6. he infamously wrote at the time: Augustine, *Confessions*, 211.

An Oral History

8. show a decline in partnered sexual activity: Debby Herbenick et al., "Changes in Penile–Vaginal Intercourse Frequency and Sexual Repertoire from 2009 to 2018: Findings from the National Survey of Sexual Health and Behavior," *Archives of Sexual Behavior* 51, no. 3 (2022): 1419–33.

8. losing the desire to place swords in sheaths: Herbenick et al., "Changes in Penile–Vaginal Intercourse."

9. numerous health benefits: Kaye Wellings et al., "Changes in, and Factors Associated with, Frequency of Sex in Britain: Evidence from Three National Surveys of Sexual Attitudes and Lifestyles (Natsal)," *British Medical Journal* 365 (2019): l1525.

9. sex *at least* once a week: "Sexual Health," National Health Service (NHS), accessed April 12, 2022, https://nhs.uk/live-well/sexual-health/.

9. oral sex was more popular than vaginal sex: Richard O. de Visser et al., "Change and Stasis in Sexual Health and Relationships: Comparisons between the First and Second Australian Studies of Health and Relationships," *Sexual Health* 11, no. 5 (2014): 505–9, https://doi.org/10.1071/SH14112.

11. receiving oral sex was even worse: Archbishop Theodore of Canterbury, "Early Penitentials: The Canons of Theodore," Internet Archive, accessed April 12, 2022, https://archive.org/details /EarlyPenitentialsTheCanonsOfTheodore/mode/2up.

13. receiving oral sex was not classified as *sex*: Peter Tiersma, "The Language of Perjury," accessed April 14, 2022, http://languageandlaw.org/PERJURY.HTM.

13. what is sex: Stephanie A. Sanders and June Machover Reinisch, "Would You Say You 'Had Sex' If . . . ?," *Journal of the American Medical Association* 281, no. 3 (1999): 275–77.

13. "soaking" in the young Mormon community: Dee Salmin, "What Is 'Soaking'—the Mormon Sex Practise That's Gone Viral on TikTok?," *ABC News*, October 5, 2021, https://abc.net.au/triplej /programs/the-hook-up/soaking-mormon-sex-tiktok-viral-jump-humping/13572802.

14. oral sex constituted having sex: Richard O. de Visser et al., "Attitudes toward Sex and Relationships: The Second Australian Study of Health and Relationships," *Sexual Health* 11, no. 5 (2014): 397–405.

Rimming: Talking in Tongues

16. Rates of anal sex: Richard O. de Visser et al., "Change and Stasis in Sexual Health and Relationships: Comparisons between the First and Second Australian Studies of Health and Relationships," *Sexual Health* 11, no. 5 (2014): 505–9, https://doi.org/10.1071/SH14112.

16. Rimming is on the rise: Tiffany R. Phillips et al., "Oral, Vaginal and Anal Sexual Practices among Heterosexual Males and Females Attending a Sexual Health Clinic: A Cross-Sectional Survey in Melbourne, Australia," *International Journal of Environmental Research and Public Health* 18, no. 23 (2021): 12668.

17. visually, it is omnipresent: Erik Wade (@erik_kaars), "THREAD: So I study medieval sex, and what *fascinates* me are sex acts that don't get discussed in medieval texts," Twitter, September 26, 2020, 7:17 a.m., https://twitter.com/erik_kaars/status/1309859549311127552?lang=en.

17. backside was associated with filth: Martha Bayless, *Sin and Filth in Medieval Culture: The Devil in the Latrine* (New York: Routledge, 2012), 17.

17. bum-kissing even became associated with witchcraft: Rosemary Ellen Guiley, *The Encyclopedia of Witches, Witchcraft and Wicca* (New York: Facts on File, 2010), 192.

18. rimming was so deeply rooted in sin: Jonathan Riley-Smith, *The Oxford Illustrated History of the Crusades* (Oxford, UK: Oxford University Press, 1995), 213.

18. **who is that seeking entry to the dining room:** Michael Kelly and Theodore Edward Hook, *Reminiscences of Michael Kelly, of the King's Theatre, and Theatre Royal Drury Lane, Including a Period of Nearly Half a Century*, vol. 1 (London: H. Colburn, 1826), 226.

20. **Mozart was undoubtedly an ass man:** Alan Dundes, *Life Is like a Chicken Coop Ladder: A Study of German National Character through Folklore* (Detroit: Wayne State University Press, 1984), 66.

20. **letters contained some kind of poo joke:** *Mozart's Letters, Mozart's Life*, ed. and trans. Robert Spaethling (New York: W. W. Norton, 2000), 87.

20. **pornographic novels, such as *120 Days of Sodom*:** Marquis de Sade, *120 Days of Sodom*, trans. James Havoc (Sun Vision Press, 2012), 78.

20. **"If it is the dirty element that gives pleasure":** Marquis de Sade, *Juliette*, trans. Austryn Wainhouse (New York: Grove Press, 1968), 26.

21. **"sinful" licking of all kinds:** Phillips et al., "Oral, Vaginal and Anal Sexual Practices."

Sense and Syphilis

22. **six people to sing "Lick Me in the Arse":** Allan Kozinn, "Three Naughty Mozart Texts Are Found," *New York Times*, March 2, 1991.

22. **abortion and infanticide:** Joseph G. Schenker and V. Rabenou, "Contraception: Traditional and Religious Attitudes," *European Journal of Obstetrics, Gynecology, and Reproductive Biology* 49, no. 1–2 (1993): 15–18.

22. **ideas regarding how to prevent pregnancy:** Paul Chrystal, *In Bed with the Ancient Greeks* (Gloucestershire, UK: Amberley, 2016), 112.

23. **weight gain to prevent any unwanted pregnancies:** Schenker and Rabenou, "Contraception."

23. **vigorous movement as a means for anti-conception:** Soranus, *Soranus' Gynecology*, trans. Owsei Temkin (Baltimore: Johns Hopkins Press, 1956), 61.

23. **Other contraceptive methods are listed:** Charlotte Booth, *In Bed with the Ancient Egyptians* (Gloucestershire, UK: Amberley, 2015), 204.

23. **one that was likely somewhat successful:** Richard G. Lipsey, Kenneth I. Carlaw, and Clifford T. Bekar, "Historical Record on the Control of Family Size," in *Economic Transformations: General Purpose Technologies and Long-Term Economic Growth* (Oxford, UK: Oxford University Press, 2005), 335–40.

24. **regarding whether early condoms can be traced:** Aine Collier, *The Humble Little Condom: A History* (Buffalo, NY: Prometheus Books, 2007), 371.

24. **The only male contraceptives recorded reliably:** J. Toivari-Viitala, *Women at Deir el-Medina:*

A Study of the Status and Roles of the Female Inhabitants in the Workmen's Community during the Ramesside Period (Leiden: Nederlands Instituut voor het Nabije Oosten, 2001), 168.

24. "foot of a female weasel": B. E. Finch and Hugh Green, *Contraception through the Ages* (London: Peter Owen, 1963), 85.

24. "two testicles of a weasel": "Toronto Museum Explores History of Contraceptives," *ABC News*, August 12, 2003, https://abc.net.au/news/2003-08-13/toronto-museum-explores-history-of -contraceptives/1463884.

24. syphilis was far more deadly: Jared Diamond, *Guns, Germs, and Steel* (New York: W. W. Norton, 1997), 210.

24. uses of condoms simultaneously appear: Y. Scott Matsumoto, Akira Koizumi, and Tadahiro Nohara, "Condom Use in Japan," *Studies in Family Planning* 3, no. 10 (1972): 251–55.

25. linen sheaths that were soaked in a chemical: H. Youssef, "The History of the Condom," *Journal of the Royal Society of Medicine* 86, no. 4 (1993): 226–28.

25. widespread syphilis epidemic: Simon Szreter and Kevin Siena, "The Pox in Boswell's London: An Estimate of the Extent of Syphilis Infection in the Metropolis in the 1770s," *Economic History Review* 74, no. 2 (2020): 372–99.

25. number of Londoners who contracted gonorrhea: University of Cambridge, "One in Five Georgian Londoners Had Syphilis by Their Mid-30s," *ScienceDaily*, July 26, 2020, www.sciencedaily .com/releases/2020/07/200706113937.htm.

25. The spread of syphilis and the popularity: Szreter and Siena, "The Pox in Boswell's London."

26. "condoms designed for gentlemen": Richard Gordon, *The Alarming History of Medicine* (New York: St. Martin's Press, 1994), 144.

26. "implements of safety": Mrs. Phillips, "Mrs. Phillips [. . .] Machine Warehouse [. . .]: She Likewise Has Great Choice of Skins and Bladders," Lisa Unger Baskin Collection, Rubenstein Rare Book and Manuscript Library, Duke University, accessed May 2, 2023, https://exhibits.library.duke .edu/exhibits/show/baskin/item/4441.

Lord of the Pills

27. activity outside marriage had been skyrocketing: Gordon Carmichael, "Non-marital Pregnancy and the Second Demographic Transition in Australia in Historical Perspective," *Demographic Research* 30, no. 21 (2014): 609–40.

28. "After 15 years": "UF Study: Sexual Revolution Began with 'Silent Generation' of '40s and '50s," University of Florida News, November 29, 2004, https://news.ufl.edu/archive/2004/11/uf-study -sexual-revolution-began-with-silent-generation-of-40s-and-50s.html.

28. data from symptomatic outcomes: Beth Bailey, *Sex in the Heartland* (Cambridge, MA: Harvard University Press, 1999), 24.

28. National Venereal Disease Control Act: Bailey, *Sex in the Heartland*, 24.

28. rising rates of horniness: Alfred C. Kinsey, *Sexual Behavior in the Human Female* (Philadelphia: W. B. Saunders, 1953).

29. exactly what they sound like: John D'Emilio and Estelle B. Freedman, *Intimate Matters: A History of Sexuality in America* (Chicago: University of Chicago Press, 1997), 257.

Living in Sin

30. dinner party will become quite rowdy: Marianna Hunt, "Party Tricks and Naked Writing: The Eccentric Life of Victor Hugo," *Guardian*, December 30, 2018, https://theguardian .com/books/booksblog/2018/dec/30/party-tricks-and-naked-writing-the-eccentric-life-of-victor -hugo.

30. He boasted in his diaries: Edward Behr, *Les Misérables: History in the Making* (London: Jonathan Cape, 1989), 14.

30. Foucher was far: Kathryn M. Grossman, *The Early Novels of Victor Hugo: Toward a Poetics of Harmony* (Geneva: Librairie Droz, 1986), 160.

31. marriage is the ultimate cockblock: Kaye Wellings et al., "Changes in, and Factors Associated with, Frequency of Sex in Britain: Evidence from Three National Surveys of Sexual Attitudes and Lifestyles (Natsal)," *British Medical Journal* 365 (2019): l1525.

31. living with someone leads to more sex: Bob Erens et al., *National Survey of Sexual Attitudes and Lifestyles II: Reference Tables and Summary Report* (2003), 111.

31. Hugo, however, was not overly fazed: Leslie Smith Dow, *Adèle Hugo: La Misérable* (Fredericton, NB: Goose Lane, 1993), 26.

31. his sex timetable: Irving Wallace, *The Intimate Sex Lives of Famous People* (Port Townsend, WA: Feral House, 2008), 166.

32. dating is now: "Dating Services—Australia," Statista, accessed May 2, 2023, https://statista .com/outlook/dmo/eservices/dating-services/australia.

Love and Friends (with Benefits)

37. term "free love": Lawrence Foster, "Free Love and Community: John Humphrey Noyes and the Oneida Perfectionists," in *America's Communal Utopias*, ed. Donald E. Pitzer (Chapel Hill: University of North Carolina Press, 1997), 253–78.

37. community practiced "complex marriage": Gregory Claeys and Lyman Tower Sargent, *The Utopia Reader*, 2nd ed. (New York: New York University Press, 2017), 217–19.

37. idea of "male continence": Heather M. Van Wormer, "The Ties That Bind: Ideology, Material Culture, and the Utopian Ideal," *Historical Archaeology* 40, no. 1 (2006): 37–56.

38. biologically inclined toward nonmonogamy: "Sexual Conflict in Human Mating | David Buss | TEDxVienna," YouTube video, 18:59, posted by TEDx Talks, November 14, 2017, https://youtube.com/watch?v=mu4Uki8VyLc.

38. cheating is going out of fashion: Richard O. de Visser et al., "Change and Stasis in Sexual Health and Relationships: Comparisons between the First and Second Australian Studies of Health and Relationships," *Sexual Health* 11, no. 5 (2014): 505–9, https://doi.org/10.1071/SH14112.

39. polyamory and open relationships: Heather Kelly, "Google's Top Searches for 2017: Matt Lauer, Hurricane Irma and More," CNN Business, December 13, 2017, https://money.cnn.com/2017/12/13/technology/google-top-searches-2017/index.html.

40. relational well-being had more influence: Jessica Wood et al., "Reasons for Sex and Relational Outcomes in Consensually Nonmonogamous and Monogamous Relationships: A Self-Determination Theory Approach," *Journal of Social and Personal Relationships* 35, no. 4 (2018), 650.

41. not a concept of which Einstein thought: Patrick J. Kiger, "Genius Albert Einstein's Theory of Infidelity," *National Geographic*, accessed May 2, 2023, https://www.natgeotv.com/za/special/genius-albert-einsteins-theory-of-infidelity.

41. humans were not meant to be monogamous: Kiger, "Genius Albert Einstein's Theory of Infidelity."

41. wives were expected to passively accept: Kiger, "Genius Albert Einstein's Theory of Infidelity."

42. A list of conditions: Kiger, "Genius Albert Einstein's Theory of Infidelity."

42. he did not stick to the rule that he'd laid out: Kiger, "Genius Albert Einstein's Theory of Infidelity."

A Degree of One's Own

43. one of the many unexpected environmental: Juliet Richters et al., "Masturbation, Paying for Sex, and Other Sexual Activities: The Second Australian Study of Health and Relationships," *Sexual Health* 11, no. 5 (2014): 461–71.

43. increase in the number of sexual partners: David Spiegelhalter, *Sex by Numbers* (London: Profile Books, 2015), 30.

43. university is also associated with homosexuality: Andrew E. Grulich et al., "Homosexual Experience and Recent Homosexual Encounters: The Second Australian Study of Health and Relationships," *Sexual Health* 11, no. 5 (2014): 439–50.

44. nothing more orgasmically powerful: Richard O. de Visser et al., "Change and Stasis in Sexual Health and Relationships: Comparisons between the First and Second Australian Studies of Health and Relationships," *Sexual Health* 11, no. 5 (2014): 505–9, https://doi.org/10.1071/SH14112.

44. statistically, you should sleep with a woman: Chris Rissel et al., "Heterosexual Experience and Recent Heterosexual Encounters among Australian Adults: The Second Australian Study of Health and Relationships," *Sexual Health* 11, no. 5 (2014): 416–26.

44. numbers of sexual partners: Spiegelhalter, *Sex by Numbers*, 31.

45. There is some sign of this gap closing: Michelle G. Alexander and Terri D. Fisher, "Truth and Consequences: Using the Bogus Pipeline to Examine Sex Differences in Self-Reported Sexuality," *Journal of Sex Research* 40, no. 1 (2003): 27–35.

46. Sex workers are often not included: Spiegelhalter, *Sex by Numbers*, 34.

46. culture of liberality that defines: Grulich et al., "Homosexual Experience and Recent Homosexual Encounters."

THE PLEASURE KINK

50. enjoy the five-finger shuffle: Juliet Richters et al., "Masturbation, Paying for Sex, and Other Sexual Activities: The Second Australian Study of Health and Relationships," *Sexual Health* 11, no. 5 (2014): 461–71.

50. social role masturbation is believed: Paul Chrystal, *In Bed with the Ancient Greeks* (Gloucestershire, UK: Amberley, 2016), 91.

51. eating in public was likely considered as taboo: Chrystal, *In Bed with the Ancient Greeks*, 92.

The War on Masturbation: One Hundred Hands of Solitude

53. phrases we use to describe masturbation: Kate Lister, *A Curious History of Sex* (London: Unbound, 2020), 25.

54. invented to stop people from masturbating: John Harvey Kellogg, *Plain Facts for Old and Young: Embracing the Natural History and Hygiene of Organic Life* (Burlington, IA: Segner, 1887), https://wellcomecollection.org/works/sbjyrqhy.

55. anti-masturbatory attitudes have continued: David Spiegelhalter, *Sex by Numbers* (London: Profile Books, 2015), 105.

55. historical statistics regarding the practice: Spiegelhalter, *Sex by Numbers*, 110.

55. resulting physical and spiritual ailments: Katharine Davis, *Factors in the Sex Life of Twenty-Two Hundred Women* (New York: Harper and Brothers, 1929).

55. many men still feared mental illness: W. H. Masters and V. E. Johnson, *Human Sexual Response* (Toronto and New York: Bantam Books, 1966).

55. How we talk and think about self-pleasure: Spiegelhalter, *Sex by Numbers*, 115.

56. recorded participants in the act of self-love: Masters and Johnson, *Human Sexual Response*.

57. Masters and Johnson became notorious: Thomas Maier, *Masters of Sex: The Life and Times of William Masters and Virginia Johnson, the Couple Who Taught America How to Love* (New York: Basic Books, 2009).

57. Masters and Johnson had a profound impact: Susan Ekberg Stiritz and Susan Frelich Appleton, "Celebrating Masters & Johnson's Human Sexual Response: A Washington University Legacy in Limbo," *Washington University Journal of Law and Policy* 53 (2017): 65–67.

The Birth of the Dildo

58. phallic batons: Hallie Lieberman, *Buzz: The Stimulating History of the Sex Toy* (New York: Simon and Schuster, 2017), 20.

59. dildos played a starring role: Paul Chrystal, *In Bed with the Ancient Greeks* (Gloucestershire, UK: Amberley, 2016), 90.

59. The penis was highly symbolic: Chrystal, *In Bed with the Ancient Greeks*, 164.

59. Aphrodite's temple: Chrystal, *In Bed with the Ancient Greeks*, 165.

60. Aristophanes's comedy *Lysistrata*: Aristophanes, *Lysistrata*, trans. George Theodoridis (2000), 1:1.110.

61. go against the grain: Peter James and Nick Thorpe, *Ancient Inventions* (New York: Ballantine Books, 1995) 183–84.

61. This has been called an *olisbokollix*: *Oxford English Dictionary*, s.v. "olisbos," accessed May 18, 2022, https://oed.com/view/Entry/131092?redirectedFrom=olisbos.

61. richly complicated lexicon: Vicki León, *The Joy of Sexus: Lust, Love, and Longing in the Ancient World* (London: Walker, 2013), 169.

61. olive oil was generously smeared on dildos: Chrystal, *In Bed with the Ancient Greeks*, 165.

62. oldest literary reference on record of the dildo: Jewish Publication Society, *Tanakh: The Holy Scriptures; The New JPS Translation According to the Traditional Hebrew Text* (Philadelphia: Jewish Publication Society, 1985).

63. dildos were also used as funerary objects: Claire Voon, "From a Jade Suit to Bronze Dildos, Ancient Tomb Luxuries of the Han Dynasty Elite," *Hyperallergic*, March 28, 2017, https://

hyperallergic.com/367055/from-a-jade-suit-to-bronze-dildos-ancient-tomb-luxuries-of-the-han
-dynasty-elite/.

63. not merely for decorative purposes: Alexandra Klausner, "The Ancient Chinese Were Pretty Kinky," *New York Post*, January 26, 2017, https://nypost.com/2017/01/26/the-ancient-chinese-were
-pretty-kinky/.

64. "Then he uncovered his basket": Pietro Aretino, *The Ragionamenti, or Dialogues of the Divine Pietro Aretino*, trans. Mark Antony Raimondi (Paris: Isidore Liseux, 1889), 14–15.

65. ejaculating dildos: Science Museum Group, "Ivory Dildo, Possibly French, 1701–1800," accessed October 2022, https://collection.sciencemuseumgroup.org.uk/objects/co8421549/ivory
-dildo-possibly-French-1701-1800-dildos-sexual-aids-penises.

65. traveling dildo salesman: William Shakespeare, *The Winter's Tale* (London: William Collins, 2013), 190–98.

66. a dildo of "thick congealed glasse": Shakespeare, *Winter's Tale*, 272–23.

66. link the dildo to anxieties of emasculation: Shakespeare, *Winter's Tale*, 98–99.

67. Mistress Frances lends a "helping hand": Shakespeare, *Winter's Tale*, 131–32.

68. singing the praises of the dildo: Shakespeare, *Winter's Tale*, 237–44.

68. rakish libertine at the other end of the table: John Wilmot, *The Complete Poems of John Wilmot, Earl of Rochester*, ed. David M. Vieth (New Haven, CT: Yale University Press, 1968).

68. large order of dildos: James William Johnson, *A Profane Wit: The Life of John Wilmot, Earl of Rochester* (Rochester, NY: University of Rochester Press, 2004), 104.

69. why an Italian lover: Jack Holland, *A Brief History of Misogyny: The World's Oldest Prejudice* (London: Castle and Robinson, 2006), 154.

69. laws were written to ban women: Lieberman, *Buzz*, 20.

70. notable variety of dildos: Allan H. Mankoff, *Mankoff's Lusty Europe* (New York: Viking, 1972).

70. safe penile substitute: Lieberman, *Buzz*, 94.

Definitions of Pleasure

72. "womansplaining themselves": Katharine Davis, *Factors in the Sex Life of Twenty-Two Hundred Women* (New York: Harper and Brothers, 1929).

72. two people reported that they had ever self-pleasured: Simon Szreter and Kate Fisher, *Sex before the Sexual Revolution: Intimate Life in England 1918–1963* (Cambridge, UK: Cambridge University Press, 2010).

72. increased sexual activity in women: M. Gerressu et al., "Prevalence of Masturbation and Associated Factors in a British National Probability Survey," *Archives of Sexual Behavior* 37, no. 2 (2008): 266–78.

The Pleasure Principle

74. circular model of women's sexual responses: Aleksandar Damjanović, Dragana Duišin, and Jasmina Barišić, "The Evolution of the Female Sexual Response Concept: Treatment Implications," *Srpski Arhiv za Celokupno Lekarstvo* 141, no. 3–4 (2013), 268–74.

74. another circular model: Heather L. Armstrong, *Encyclopedia of Sex and Sexuality: Understanding Biology, Psychology, and Culture*, 2 vols. (London: Bloomsbury, 2021), 160.

75. complexity of the woman's orgasm: "It's possible that women are genuinely less clear than men about what counts as masturbation": Juliet Richters and Chris Rissel, *Doing It Down Under: The Sexual Lives of Australians* (Crows Nest, Australia: Allen and Unwin, 2014), 39.

76. defining masturbation: Allison L. Kirschbaum and Zoë D. Peterson, "Would You Say You 'Had Masturbated' If . . . ?: The Influence of Situational and Individual Factors on Labeling a Behavior as Masturbation," *Journal of Sex Research* 55, no. 2 (2018): 263–72.

76. "masturbation does not have one universal": Kirschbaum and Peterson, "Would You Say You 'Had Masturbated.' "

The Vibrator: Good Vibes Only

78. A wandering womb: *Aretaiou Kappadokou Ta Sozomena: The Extant Works of Aretaeus, the Cappadocian*, ed. and trans. Francis Adams (London: Sydenham Society, 1856), https://wellcomecollection.org/works/d92pst4q.

79. "hysterical suffocation": Elaine Fantham et al., *Women in the Classical World: Image and Text* (New York: Oxford University Press, 1995), 199.

80. prescribed cures for female hysteria: Cecilia Tasca et al., "Women and Hysteria in the History of Mental Health," *Clinical Practice and Epidemiology in Mental Health* 8 (2012): 110–19.

80. woman's hysteria would be cured for good: Rachel Maines, *The Technology of Orgasm: "Hysteria," the Vibrator, and Women's Sexual Satisfaction* (Baltimore: Johns Hopkins University Press, 1999).

80. stimulation of the area with oils and scents: Winifried Schleiner, *Medical Ethics in the Renaissance* (Washington, DC: Georgetown University Press, 1995), 115.

81. hysteria more of a psychological ailment: Regina Markell Morantz and Sue Zschoche, "Professionalism, Feminism, and Gender Roles: A Comparative Study of Nineteenth-Century Medical Therapeutics," *Journal of American History* 67, no. 3 (1980): 568–88.

83. the prevalence of vibrator use by men: Michael Reece et al., "Prevalence and Characteristics of Vibrator Use by Men in the United States," *Journal of Sexual Medicine* 6, no. 7 (2009): 1867–74.

84. any areas of titillating stimulation: James Craven Wood, *Clinical Gynecology* (Philadelphia: Boericke and Tafel, 1917), 21.

84. Bodysex workshops: Betty Dodson, *Sex for One: The Joy of Self-Loving* (New York: Crown Trade, 1996), 154.

85. effects of different masturbation techniques: S. McMullen and R. C. Rosen, "Self-Administered Masturbation Training in the Treatment of Primary Orgasmic Dysfunction," *Journal of Consulting and Clinical Psychology* 47, no. 5 (1979): 912–18.

85. success using the Betty Dodson Method: Pia Struck and Søren Ventegodt, "Clinical Holistic Medicine: Teaching Orgasm for Females with Chronic Anorgasmia Using the Betty Dodson Method," *Scientific World Journal* 8 (2008): 883–95.

85. this wand's newfound magic: Cathy Winks and Anne Semans, *The New Good Vibrations Guide to Sex: Tips and Techniques from America's Favorite Sex Toy Store* (Jersey City, NJ: Cleis Press, 1997), 102, 154.

86. "phallic fantasy": Susan Ekberg Stiritz and Susan Frelich Appleton, "Celebrating Masters & Johnson's Human Sexual Response: A Washington University Legacy in Limbo," *Washington University Journal of Law and Policy* 53 (2017): 65–67.

86. some of the bestselling sex toys today: "Retail Sales Value Share of the Sexual Wellness Devices Market Worldwide in 2021, by Product Category," Statista, December 1, 2021, https://statista.com/statistics/1349370/sex-toys-market-by-product-category/.

(Self) Love in Lockdown

87. The use of sex toys has been on the rise: Richard O. de Visser et al., "Change and Stasis in Sexual Health and Relationships: Comparisons between the First and Second Australian Studies of Health and Relationships," *Sexual Health* 11, no. 5 (2014): 505–9, https://doi.org/10.1071/SH14112.

87. sex-toy sales skyrocketed: Alexandra Hourigan, "Love in Lockdown: 14% of Aussies Are No Longer Meeting New Partners, so Here's How You Can Scratch That Itch," Finder, August 17, 2021, https://finder.com.au/love-in-lockdown-picks.

87. We-Vibe claimed a 180 percent increase in sales: Patrick Tadros, "Sex Toy Sales Are Buzzing during COVID-19 Pandemic," *Daily Telegraph*, October 6, 2021.

89. brings us to ben wa balls: Hallie Lieberman, *Buzz: The Stimulating History of the Sex Toy* (New York: Simon and Schuster, 2017), 25.

89. *Rin no tama* were adopted by sex workers: Lieberman, *Buzz*, 25.

QUEER KINKS

93. **The usual culprits—Woolf, Joyce, and Fitzgerald:** Quote adapted from Woolf's diaries, recounting her first meeting with Freud at her house. Original quote: "Dr. Freud gave me a narcissus. Was sitting in a great library with little statues at a large scrupulously tidy shiny table. We like patients on chairs. A screwed up shrunk very old man: with a monkey's light eyes, paralyzed spasmodic movements, inarticulate: but alert." Virginia Woolf, *The Diary of Virginia Woolf*, ed. Anne Oliver Bell and Andrew McNeillie, vol. 5, *1936–1941* (New York: Harvest Books, 1986), 202.

93. **"If you read Freud":** Virginia Woolf, "Character in Fiction (1924)," in *The Essays of Virginia Woolf*, ed. A. McNeillie, vol. 3, *1919–1924*, appendix 3 (London: Hogarth Press, 1988), 504.

94. **"has *everything* to do with sex":** Jeri Johnson, introduction to *The Psychology of Love*, by Sigmund Freud, trans. Shaun Whiteside (Melbourne, Australia: Penguin Books, 2010), xxiii.

95. **"gender or sexual fluidity":** Fern Riddell, *Sex: Lessons from History* (London: Hodder and Stoughton, 2021), 35.

Language and Labels: What's in a Name?

98. **only 1.3 percent of men:** Juliet Richters et al., "Sexual Identity, Sexual Attraction and Sexual Experience: The Second Australian Study of Health and Relationships," *Sexual Health* 11, no. 5 (2014): 451–60.

99. **homoerotic *behavior* to homosexual *identification*:** Rebecca S. Geary et al., "Sexual Identity, Attraction and Behaviour in Britain: The Implications of Using Different Dimensions of Sexual Orientation to Estimate the Size of Sexual Minority Populations and Inform Public Health Interventions," *PloS One* 13, no. 1 (2018): e0189607.

101. **"We call these people bisexual":** Sigmund Freud, *Analysis Terminable and Interminable* (London: Hogarth Press, 1964), 261.

102. **Freud's work has been entirely disregarded:** Frederick Crews, "The Verdict on Freud," *Psychological Science* 7, no. 2 (1996), 63–68.

Orlando: A Bi-ography

103. **no other sexuality that has been so heavily:** Philip W. Blumstein and Pepper Schwartz, "Lesbianism and Bisexuality," in *Sexual Deviance and Sexual Deviants*, ed. Erich Goode (New York: William Morrow, 1974), 78–295; Thomas Geller, ed., *Bisexuality: A Reader and Sourcebook* (Novato, CA: Times Change Press, 1990); Paula C. Rust, "When Does the Unity of a 'Common Oppression' Break Down? Reciprocal Attitudes between Lesbian and Bisexual Women" (PhD diss., University of Michigan, 1989).

An Asexual History

110. Andersen kept a meticulous journal: Jackie Wullschläger, *Hans Christian Andersen: The Life of a Storyteller* (New York: A. A. Knopf, 2001), 70.

111. unnerved by the thought of sexual interaction: Hans Christian Andersen, *The Stories of Hans Christian Andersen*, trans. Diana Crone Frank and Jeffrey Frank (Boston and New York: Houghton Mifflin, 2003), 10.

111. Andersen became so scared: Andersen, *Stories of Hans Christian Andersen*, 10.

111. bounds of conventional friendship: *Hans Christian Andersen's Correspondence*, ed. Frederick Crawford (London: Dean and Son, 1891).

112. Ariel does not get a happy ending: Hans Christian Andersen, *The Little Mermaid*, trans. H. B. Paul (Hythloday Press, 2014).

112. misconceptions about asexuality: Michael Waters, "Finding Asexuality in the Archives," *Slate*, March 6, 2020.

113. "no socio-sexual contacts or reactions": Alfred C. Kinsey, Wardell B. Pomeroy, and Clyde E. Martin, *Sexual Behavior in the Human Male* (Philadelphia: W. B. Saunders, 1948).

113. 0.5 percent: Anthony F. Bogaert, "The Demography of Asexuality," in *International Handbook on the Demography of Sexuality*, ed. Amanda K. Baumle (Netherlands: Springer, 2013), 275–88.

113. 3.3 percent: Jannike Höglund et al., "Finnish Women and Men Who Self-Report No Sexual Attraction in the Past 12 Months: Prevalence, Relationship Status, and Sexual Behavior History," *Archives of Sexual Behavior* 43, no. 5 (2014): 879–89.

113. J. M. Barrie: Nico Lllewelyn Davies, interview in the introduction to Andrew Birkin, *J. M. Barrie and the Lost Boys: The Real Story Behind Peter Pan* (New Haven, CT: Yale University Press, 2003).

113. George Bernard Shaw: Michiko Kakutani, "G. B. Shaw and the Women in His Life and Art," *New York Times*, September 27, 1981.

Codes and Symbols: Somewhere over the Rainbow

114. "friend of Dorothy": James Deutsch, "Are You a Friend of Dorothy? Folk Speech of the LGBTQ Community," *Smithsonian*, June 29, 2021, https://smithsonianmag.com/blogs/smithsonian-center -folklife-cultural-heritage/2021/06/.

115. Judy Garland: Richard Dyer, *Heavenly Bodies: Film Stars and Society* (London: British Film Institute, 1986), 156.

115. In the original writings: Lyman Frank Baum, *Dorothy and the Wizard in Oz* (Chicago: Reilly and Britton, 1908).

117. all the various prior definitions of *gay*: Gertrude Stein, *Selected Writings of Gertrude Stein* (New York: Vintage Books, 1990), 563.

118. Magnus Hirschfeld: David Spiegelhalter, *Sex by Numbers* (London: Profile Books, 2015), 76.

118. human tolerance and empathy: Fern Riddell, *Sex: Lessons from History* (London: Hodder and Stoughton, 2021), 104.

118. "sexual intermediaries": Spiegelhalter, *Sex by Numbers*, 77.

118. heightened suicide rates: Heike Bauer, *The Hirschfeld Archives: Violence, Death, and Modern Queer Culture* (Philadelphia: Temple University Press, 2017).

118. the first gender-correction surgery: Riddell, *Sex*, 106.

119. passes for "transvestite" individuals: Riddell, *Sex*, 107.

A Tale of Two Sexes

120. skeleton of a "man" buried in Prague: Abigail Hudson, "LGBTQIA+ History Month—Burying the Truth: Gender, the Media, and Accessing the Past," University of Birmingham, February 11, 2021, https://blog.bham.ac.uk/historybham/lgbtqia-history-month-burying-the-truth-gender-the-media-and-accessing-the-past/.

120. did not conform to the woman/man binary: M. D. Danti and Megan Cifarelli, "Iron II Warrior Burials at Hasanlu Tepe, Iran," *Iranica Antiqua* 50 (2015): 61–157.

120. Roman emperor Elagabalus: Eric R. Varner, "Transcending Gender: Assimilation, Identity, and Roman Imperial Portraits," *Memoirs of the American Academy in Rome: Supplementary Volumes* 7 (2008): 200–201.

121. "When Zoticus addressed the emperor": Varner, "Transcending Gender."

121. Many consider Julius Caesar: Paul Chrystal, *In Bed with the Romans* (Gloucestershire, UK: Amberley, 2017), 139.

121. allowing himself to be penetrated: Dio Cassius, *Roman History*, vol. 4, book 43 (London: Heinemann, 1916), 246.

123. François-Timoléon de Choisy: Peter Wagner, *Eros Revived: Erotica of the Enlightenment in England and America* (London: Paladin, 1990), 33.

123. 1932 publication: *Airdrie & Coatbridge Advertiser*, Saturday, April 30, 1932, sourced from Fern Riddell, *Sex: Lessons from History* (London: Hodder and Stoughton, 2021).

123. Anastasia the Patrician: Randy P. Conner, David Hatfield Sparks, and Mariya Sparks, *Cassell's*

Encyclopedia of Queer Myth, Symbol and Spirit: Gay, Lesbian, Bisexual and Transgender Lore (London: UNKNO, 1998), 57.

124. reference to a third gender: Stephen O. Murray and Will Roscoe, *Islamic Homosexualities: Culture, History, and Literature* (New York: New York University Press, 1997).

124. ancient Indian culture: Peter A. Jackson, "Non-normative Sex/Gender Categories in the Theravada Buddhist Scriptures," *Australian Humanities Review* (1996).

124. five different manifestations of gender ambiguity: Mehrdad Alipour, "Islamic Shari'a Law, Neotraditionalist Muslim Scholars and Transgender Sex-Reassignment Surgery: A Case Study of Ayatollah Khomeini's and Sheikh al-Tantawi's Fatwas," *International Journal of Transgenderism* 18, no. 1 (2017): 91–103.

124. Maya civilization: Matthew G. Looper, "Women-Men (and Men-Women): Classic Maya Rulers and the Third Gender," in *Ancient Maya Women*, ed. Traci Arden (Walnut Creek, CA: AltaMira Press, 2002).

124. Inca civilization: Michael J. Horswell, "Transculturating Tropes of Sexuality, Tinkuy, and Third Gender in the Andes," in *Decolonizing the Sodomite: Queer Tropes of Sexuality in Colonial Andean Culture* (Austin: University of Texas Press, 2006).

125. performance of this castration: Chrystal, *In Bed with the Romans*, 141.

125. early example of transgender people: Kirsten Cronn-Mills, *Transgender Lives: Complex Stories, Complex Voices* (Minneapolis: Twenty-First Century Books, 2014), 39.

125. outside a dichotomy of male and female: Jacob Latham, " 'Fabulous Clap-Trap': Roman Masculinity, the Cult of Magna Mater, and Literary Constructions of the Galli at Rome from the Late Republic to Late Antiquity," *Journal of Religion* 92, no. 1 (2012): 84–122.

125. Māhū were a third-gendered people: Aleardo Zanghellini, "Sodomy Laws and Gender Variance in Tahiti and Hawai'i," *Laws* 2, no. 2 (2013): 51–68.

126. begin to be reclaimed: Carol E. Robertson, "The Māhū of Hawai'i," *Feminist Studies* 15, no. 2 (1989): 318.

126. Muxe people in the Zapotec cultures: Beverly Chiñas, "Isthmus Zapotec Attitudes toward Sex and Gender Anomalies," in *Latin American Male Homosexualities*, ed. Stephen O. Murray (Albuquerque: University of New Mexico Press, 1995), 293–302.

126. The enforcement of Christian teaching: Lynn Stephen, "Sexualities and Genders in Zapotec Oaxaca," *Latin American Perspectives* 29, no. 2 (2002): 41–59.

126. Isthmus Zapotec community were Muxe: David Rymph, "Cross-Sex Behavior in an Isthmus Zapotec Village" (paper presented at the annual meeting of the American Anthropological Association, Mexico City, 1974).

Gender Troubles: The Bluest Dress

128. **"The generally accepted rule is pink":** Jeanne Maglaty, "When Did Girls Start Wearing Pink?," *Smithsonian*, April 7, 2011, https://www.smithsonianmag.com/arts-culture/when-did-girls -start-wearing-pink-1370097.

129. **the policing of "gendered clothing":** Randolph Trumbach, "Erotic Fantasy and Male Libertinism in Enlightenment England," in *The Invention of Pornography*, ed. Lynn Hunt (New York: Zone Books, 1993), 257.

129. **women were regarded as the more sexually:** Trumbach, "Erotic Fantasy," 256.

130. **homoeroticism played a rather prominent role:** Trumbach, "Erotic Fantasy," 254–55.

130. **pederasty was a homoerotic relationship:** Paul Chrystal, *In Bed with the Ancient Greeks* (Gloucestershire, UK: Amberley, 2016), 100.

131. **Failure to show these signs of affection:** Aristophanes, *Birds*, trans. Ian Johnston (Nanaimo, BC: Vancouver Island University, 2020), 140, http://johnstoniatexts.x10host.com/aristophanes /birdshtml.html.

131. **"practiced sodomy":** Chrystal, *In Bed with the Ancient Greeks*, 98.

131. **"Greek love" referred to the act of anal sex:** Chrystal, *In Bed with the Ancient Greeks*, 99.

131. **identifying homosexuality in ancient Egypt:** Charlotte Booth, *In Bed with the Ancient Egyptians* (Gloucestershire, UK: Amberley, 2015), 145.

133. **Khnumhotep and Niankhkhnum:** "Archaeologists, Feminists, and Queers: Sexual Politics in the Construction of the Past," in Pamela L. Geller and Miranda K. Stockett, eds., *Feminist Anthropology: Past, Present, and Future* (Philadelphia: University of Pennsylvania Press, 2010), 89–102.

133. **"royal confidants":** Booth, *In Bed with the Ancient Egyptians*, 159.

133. **positions that would have been considered:** Booth, *In Bed with the Ancient Egyptians*, 160.

133. **evidence of attempts to erase the wives:** Greg Reeder, "Same-Sex Desire, Conjugal Constructs, and the Tomb of Niankhkhnum and Khnumhotep," *World Archaeology* 32, no. 2 (2000): 193–208.

Metamorphoses

134. **new ways of conceptualizing sexual selves:** Alison Better and Brandy L. Simula, "How and for Whom Does Gender Matter? Rethinking the Concept of Sexual Orientation," *Sexualities* 18, no. 5–6 (2015): 665–80.

134. **"An individual's orientation":** Better and Smiula, "How and for Whom Does Gender Matter?"

135. fluid conception of sexuality: Eva Cantarella, *Bisexuality in the Ancient World*, trans. Cormac Ó Cuilleanáin, 2nd ed. (New Haven, CT: Yale University Press, 2002).

135. Spartan women began to cut their hair: Joshua J. Mark, "Spartan Women," *World History Encyclopedia*, June 14, 2021, https://worldhistory.org/article/123/spartan-women/.

136. had come from the island of Lesbos: Paul Chrystal, *In Bed with the Ancient Greeks* (Gloucestershire, UK: Amberley, 2016), 106.

137. Sappho was dismissed: Aristotle, *Rhetoric* 1398b, quoted in Chrystal, *In Bed with the Ancient Greeks*, 106.

137. "sex-mad little whore": Tatian, *Address to the Greeks*, 33, quoted in Chrystal, *In Bed with the Ancient Greeks*, 107.

137. an effort to heterosexualize her: Chrystal, *In Bed with the Ancient Greeks*, 96.

138. "drunk for about a week": F. Scott Fitzgerald, *The Great Gatsby* (London: Penguin Classics, 2000), 47.

138. "book for the New Generation": Full quote: "Gertrude Stein and Fitzgerald are very peculiar in their relation to each other. Gertrude Stein had been very much impressed by *This Side of Paradise*. She read it when it came out and before she knew any of the young American writers. She said of it that it was this book that really created for the public the new generation. She has never changed her opinion about this. She thinks this equally true of *The Great Gatsby*. She thinks Fitzgerald will be read when many of his well known contemporaries are forgotten. Fitzgerald always says that he thinks Gertrude Stein says these things just to annoy him by making him think that she means them, and he adds in his favorite way, and her doing it is the cruelest thing I ever heard." Gertrude Stein, "The Autobiography of Alice B. Toklas," in *Selected Writings of Gertrude Stein* (New York: Vintage Books, 1990), 206.

138. "who came first, Gertrude Stein or James Joyce": Full quote: "Joyce is good. He is a good writer. People like him because he is incomprehensible and anybody can understand him. But who came first, Gertrude Stein or James Joyce? Do not forget that my first great book, *Three Lives*, was published in 1908. That was long before *Ulysses*. But Joyce has done something. His influence, however, is local. Like Synge, another Irish writer, he has had his day." Stein, "Autobiography of Alice B. Toklas," 5.

138. "I hate intellectual women": Richard Ellmann, *James Joyce: New and Revised Edition* (New York: Oxford University Press, 1982), 529.

138. "the most intelligible, but also the most popular": Virginia Woolf, "Letter 1644, dated 2 June 1926," in *Selected Letters*, ed. Joanne Trautmann Banks (London: Vintage, 2008), 211.

138. "The three geniuses": Stein, "Autobiography of Alice B. Toklas."

139. LGBTQIA+ identification doubled: Jeffrey M. Jones, "LGBT Identification in U.S. Ticks Up to 7.1%," Gallup, February 17, 2022, https://news.gallup.com/poll/389792/lgbt-identification-ticks-up.aspx.

139. willingness to disclose one's identity: Tom Wilson et al., "What Is the Size of Australia's Sexual Minority Population?," *BMC Research Notes* 13, no. 535 (2020): 1–6.

THE KINK KINK

141. "While all animals have courtship rituals": Kate Lister, *A Curious History of Sex* (London: Unbound, 2020), 1.

142. A 2017 study of the Belgian population: Lien Holvoet et al., "Fifty Shades of Belgian Gray: The Prevalence of BDSM-Related Fantasies and Activities in the General Population," *Journal of Sexual Medicine* 14, no. 9 (2017): 1152–59.

142. a similar finding emerged from Czechia: Eva Jozifkova, "Sexual Arousal by Dominance and Submissiveness in the General Population: How Many, How Strongly, and Why?," *Deviant Behavior* 39, no. 9 (2018): 1229–36.

Of Humans' Bondage

145. James Joyce's letters: Brenda Maddox, "Ah Yes—but What Ever Happened to Nora's Side of the Correspondence?," *Guardian*, July 8, 2004, https://theguardian.com/uk/2004/jul/09/books.booksnews.

147. no small feat for a Galway girl: Maddox, "Ah Yes."

148. experienced the starkest rise: "Sales of Bedroom Toys in the UK Doubles during COVID-19 Lockdown," Love the Sales, April 20, 2020, https://www.lovethesales.com/press/articles/lockdown-sex-toy-boom.

148. sexual behavior during the pandemic: Justin J. Lehmiller et al., "Less Sex, but More Sexual Diversity: Changes in Sexual Behavior during the COVID-19 Coronavirus Pandemic," *Leisure Sciences* 43, no. 1–2 (2021): 295–304.

149. KinkD put out a survey: KinkD, "A New Survey Reveals Top 10 Sexual Kinks during COVID-19 Lockdown," *PR Newswire: Cision*, May 21, 2020, https://prnewswire.com/news-releases/a-new-survey-reveals-top-10-sexual-kinks-during-covid-19-lockdown-301063398.html.

149. "Unlike real-life play": KinkD, "A New Survey Reveals."

Erotic Charges

150. intense physical sensations: Jules Vivid, Eliot M. Lev, and Richard Sprott, "The Structure of Kink Identity: Four Key Themes within a World of Complexity," *Journal of Positive Sexuality* 6, no. 2 (2020), 75–85.

150. **"Kink is more important":** Vivid, Lev, and Sprott, "The Structure of Kink Identity."

151. **selecting a partner for BDSM play:** Alison Better and Brandy L. Simula, "How and for Whom Does Gender Matter? Rethinking the Concept of Sexual Orientation," *Sexualities* 18, no. 5–6 (2015), 665–80.

152. **study done by the Burnet Institute:** Angela C. Davis et al., "What Behaviors Do Young Heterosexual Australians See in Pornography? A Cross-sectional Study," *Journal of Sex Research* 55, no. 3 (2018): 310–19.

Kinky Clothing

157. **tied to explorations of homosexuality:** Lien Holvoet et al., "Fifty Shades of Belgian Gray: The Prevalence of BDSM-Related Fantasies and Activities in the General Population," *Journal of Sexual Medicine* 14, no. 9 (2017): 1152–59.

158. **less associated with its biker foundations:** Cynthia Slater was one of the main activists for women's inclusion and would be included on the Leather Hall of Fame inductees list. See Lewis Call, *BDSM in American Science Fiction and Fantasy* (New York: Palgrave Macmillan, 2013), 5.

158. **one of the most popular fetishes:** Holvoet et al., "Fifty Shades."

159. **A black market for nylons appeared:** Audra J. Wolfe, "Nylon: A Revolution in Textiles," Science History Institute, October 3, 2008, https://sciencehistory.org/distillations/nylon-a -revolution-in-textiles?page=3.

159. **Nylon stockings became one of the prime targets:** Jeffrey L. Meikle, *American Plastic: A Cultural History* (New Brunswick, NJ: Rutgers University Press, 1997).

160. **every time stocks of nylons appeared:** Susannah Handley, *Nylon: The Story of a Fashion Revolution* (Baltimore: Johns Hopkins University Press, 1999), 48.

160. **"The fetish for me is more online":** Ralph Jones, "What's the Latest with the Vajankle, the Sex Toy Shaped like a Foot?," *Vice*, February 10, 2015, https://vice.com/en/article/ppmngm/vajankle -ralph-jones.

Foot Fetishes: The Toe-Between

162. **"The foot is an erotic organ":** William A. Rossi, *The Sex Life of the Foot and Shoe* (Malabar, FL: Krieger, 1993), 1.

162. **Philostratus worships the shape:** *The Letters of Alciphron, Aelian, and Philostratus*, trans. A. R. Benner and F. H. Fobes (Cambridge, MA: Harvard University Press, 1949), 22.

162. **"would love to kiss them":** *The Letters of Alciphron*, 67.

162. "tread on me": *The Letters of Alciphron*, 21.

163. Jesus washing the feet of his disciples: John 13:1–17.

163. The coveted foot size: Amanda Foreman, "Why Footbinding Persisted in China for a Millennium," *Smithsonian*, February 2015, https://smithsonianmag.com/history/why-footbinding-persisted-china-millennium-180953971/.

164. Fitzgerald repeatedly visited one sex worker: Tony Buttitta, *The Lost Summer: A Personal Memoir of F. Scott Fitzgerald* (New York: St. Martin's Press, 1987), 41, 112–13.

164. "Freudian shame about his feet": F. Scott Fitzgerald, *Ledger: A Facsimile* (Washington, DC: NCR Microcard, 1972), 157.

164. "a bit of cross-wiring": Vilayanur S. Ramachandran and Sandra Blakeslee, *Phantoms in the Brain: Probing the Mysteries of the Human Mind* (New York: William Morrow, 1999).

165. factors that may have impacted the foot fetish: A. J. Giannini et al., "Sexualization of the Female Foot as a Response to Sexually Transmitted Epidemics: A Preliminary Study," *Psychological Reports* 83, no. 2 (1998): 491–98.

165. sexual focus on the female foot emerged: The medieval poem "The Romance of the Rose (Le Roman de la Rose)" and the work of Cerverí de Girona are quoted as examples of this.

165. the term *toe-cleavage*: Hans Rudolph Meyer, "The Female Foot," *Foot & Ankle International* 17, no. 2 (1996): 120–24.

165. safe alternative to penetrative sex: R. Williams, "Striving to Reach New Heights," *Leg Action* 12, no. 10 (1994): 3; D. Hanson, "My Opinion," *Leg Show* 13, no. 6 (1995): 4–5.

165. number of foot-oriented pictures: Giannini et al., "Sexualization of the Female Foot."

Crime and Pleasurable Punishment

168. "With opportunity for the natural satisfaction": Richard von Krafft-Ebing, *Psychopathia Sexualis: A Medico-Forensic Study* (Burlington, VT: Elsevier Science, 2013), 79.

168. use of painful activities: Frédérike Labrecque et al., "What Is So Appealing about Being Spanked, Flogged, Dominated, or Restrained? Answers from Practitioners of Sexual Masochism/Submission," *Journal of Sex Research* 58, no. 4 (2021): 409–23.

169. accidental deaths due to strangulation: Peter Wagner, *Eros Revived: Erotica of the Enlightenment in England and America* (London: Paladin, 1990), 25.

169. "An Essay on the Art of Strangulation": Wagner, *Eros Revived*, 25.

169. **strangulation was a productive way:** Wagner, *Eros Revived*, 27.

169. **consensual violence:** Angela C. Davis et al., "What Behaviors Do Young Heterosexual Australians See in Pornography?," *Journal of Sex Research* 55, no. 3 (2018): 310–19.

169. **"US population engages in sadomasochism":** June M. Reinisch, Ruth Beasley, and Debra Kent, *The Kinsey Institute New Report on Sex* (New York: St. Martin's Press, 1990), 162.

170. **human experiences of pain and pleasure:** Barry R. Komisaruk et al., "Women's Clitoris, Vagina, and Cervix Mapped on the Sensory Cortex: fMRI Evidence," *Journal of Sexual Medicine* 8, no. 10 (2011): 2822–30.

171. **toy-related injuries increased by 50 percent:** Christopher Ingraham, "Sex Toy Injuries Surged after 'Fifty Shades of Grey' Was Published," *Washington Post*, February 10, 2015, https://washingtonpost.com/news/wonk/wp/2015/02/10/sex-toy-injuries-surged-after-fifty-shades-of-grey-was-published/.

173. **"it is the sub who has all the power":** E. L. James, *Fifty Shades of Grey* (London: Arrow, 2012), 400.

173. **"the receiver (the masochist), not the giver (the sadist)":** Reinisch, Beasley, and Kent, *Kinsey Institute New Report*, 162–63.

173. **"so-called traditional sex roles are reversed":** Reinisch, Beasley, and Kent, *Kinsey Institute New Report*, 162–63.

173. **experience of many during sexual role-play:** Robin Bauer, "Transgressive and Transformative Gendered Sexual Practices and White Privileges: The Case of the Dyke/Trans BDSM Communities," *Women's Studies Quarterly* 36, no. 3–4 (2008): 233–53.

174. **performative character of gender:** Bauer, "Transgressive and Transformative Gendered Sexual Practices," 248.

175. **care of Mademoiselle Lambercier:** Jean-Jacques Rousseau, *The Confessions of J. J. Rousseau* (New York: Calvin Blanchard, 1856), 31.

175. **"determined my taste":** Rousseau, *Confessions*, 32.

175. **he found himself desirous:** Rousseau, *Confessions*, 32.

176. **awareness of his kink at an early age:** Lien Holvoet et al., "Fifty Shades of Belgian Gray: The Prevalence of BDSM-Related Fantasies and Activities in the General Population," *Journal of Sexual Medicine* 14, no. 9 (2017): 1152–59.

176. **he tried to fight his sexual desire for spanking:** Rousseau, *Confessions*, 33.

176. **intoxication of this fantasy was enough:** Rousseau, *Confessions*, 34.

177. Rousseau desired to surprise beautiful ladies: Rousseau, *Confessions*, 114.

177. he wrote an autobiographical work: Rousseau, *Confessions*, 308–9.

178. Lewis reportedly became fascinated: Alan Jacobs, *The Narnian: The Life and Imagination of C. S. Lewis* (New York: HarperCollins, 2009).

178. wrote letters to his friend Arthur Greeves: Alister McGrath, *C. S. Lewis: A Life; Eccentric Genius, Reluctant Prophet* (Carol Stream, IL: Tyndale House, 2013), 62.

The Lion, the Witch, and the Dominatrix

179. Hymns to this goddess: "Inana and Ebih: Translation," Electronic Text Corpus of Sumerian Literature, University of Oxford, http://etcsl.orinst.ox.ac.uk/section1/tr132.htm.

179. rituals of the cult members: Anne O. Nomis, *The History & Arts of the Dominatrix* (Basingstoke, UK: Anna Nomis Ltd, 2013), 53.

180. The dominatrix was born in literature: Anne Lyon Haight, ed., *Hroswitha of Gandersheim: Her Life, Times and Works, and a Comprehensive Bibliography* (New York: Hroswitha Club, 1965), 21, 42.

181. "unattainable woman": Francis X. Newman, ed., *The Meaning of Courtly Love* (Albany: State University of New York Press, 1968), vii.

181. Fantasies of cruel love and domination: Robert Herrick, *The Poetical Works of Robert Herrick*, ed. F. W. Moorman (London: Oxford University Press, 1951).

182. Berkley's establishment specialized in flagellation: Note: Ashbee does not quote the source of this statement in his writing from the 1880s. Henry Spencer Ashbee, *Index of Forbidden Books* (London: Sphere, 1969), 147; originally written in the 1880s as *Index Librorum Prohibitorum*.

182. the Berkley Horse: Ashbee, *Index of Forbidden Books*, 147.

183. let customers return the favor: Bernhardt J. Hurwood, *The Golden Age of Erotica* (Los Angeles: Sherbourne Press, 1965), 161.

183. Even nuns are guilty: Henry Thomas Buckle, *Exhibition of Female Flagellants in the Modest and Incontinent World* (London: Forgotten Books, 1963), 52, https://forgottenbooks.com/en/books /ExhibitionofFemaleFlagellantsintheModestandIncontinentWorld_10692401.

184. spanking could be a corrective for male impotence: Johann Heinrich Meibom, *A Treatise of the Use of Flogging in Venereal Affairs: Also of the Office of the Loins and Reins* (London: Curll, 1718), 34.

184. Cloaking sexually imaginative scenes: Meibom, *A Treatise of the Use of Flogging*, 34.

185. Scenes of flagellation crept into all corners: Ashbee, *Index of Forbidden Books*, xli.

185. infamous scenes of flagellation: John Cleland, *Fanny Hill: Memoirs of a Woman of Pleasure* (Ware, UK: Wordsworth Classics, 2001).

185. Fanny chooses her whipping device: Cleland, *Fanny Hill*, 161–62.

186. an unfortunate deformity of taste: Cleland, *Fanny Hill*, 161.

186. necessity to get their "little man" working: Edward Ward, *The London-Spy Compleat, in Eighteen Parts* (J. How, 1704), 32–33.

186. by virtue of their age: Cleland, *Fanny Hill*, 159.

186. There was another scandalous aspect: Cleland, *Fanny Hill*, 165.

186. *Gardens of Pleasure*: "Gardens of Pleasure: Eroticism and Sexual Aesthetics in Ancient China," Sotheby's, April 12, 2022, https://sothebys.com/en/articles/gardens-of-Pleasure-eroticism-and -sexual-aesthetics-in-ancient-china.

One Flew over the Cuckold's Nest

188. first appears in the English language in 1250: "The Owl and the Nightingale" (London: British Library and Jesus College, 1250), 1535–55.

188. a man made foolish by his wife's infidelity: Gordon Williams, *A Dictionary of Sexual Language and Imagery in Shakespearean and Stuart Literature* (London: Athlone Press, 2001), 336.

189. she will make a cuckold out of him: William Shakespeare, *Much Ado about Nothing* (Oxford, UK: Oxford University Press, 2009), act 2, scene 1, 43–44.

190. "believed himself likely to be a cuckold": Geoffrey Chaucer, "The Miller's Tale," in *The Canterbury Tales* (Oxford, UK: Oxford University Press, 2011), lines 113–24.

190. Titania has learned her lesson: William Shakespeare, *A Midsummer Night's Dream* (Oxford, UK: Oxford University Press, 2008), act 4, scene 1.

191. "horn-mad": Shakespeare, *Much Ado about Nothing*, act 1, scene 1, 210–11.

193. "male fear" was the ingredient: Sarah Laskow, "Everything You've Heard about Chastity Belts Is a Lie," *Atlas Obscura*, July 12, 2017, https://atlasobscura.com/articles/everything-youve-heard -about-chastity-belts-is-a-lie.

193. "curiosities for the prurient, or as jokes for the tasteless": Albrecht Classen, *The Medieval Chastity Belt: A Myth-Making Process* (London: Palgrave Macmillan, 2007), 107.

THE PORN KINK

200. pornography views rose so drastically: Paul J. Maginn, "Denied Intimacy in 'Iso,' Aussies Go Online for Adult Content—So What's Hot in Each Major City?" *The Conversation*, May 19, 2020, https://theconversation.com/denied-intimacy-in-iso-aussies-go-online-for-adult-content-so-whats-hot-in-each-major-city-138122.

200. countries who most frequently visit Pornhub: "Pornhub Has Revealed Exactly How Australians Watch Their Porn," *Men's Health Australia*, May 1, 2021, https://menshealth.com.au/exactly-how-australians-watch-porn/.

201. rates of lifetime exposure to pornography: Alan McKee, "Does Pornography Harm Young People?," *Australian Journal of Communication* 37, no. 1 (2010): 17–36.

201. median age for viewing pornography: Megan S. C. Lim et al., "Young Australians' Use of Pornography and Associations with Sexual Risk Behaviours," *Australian and New Zealand Journal of Public Health* 41, no. 4 (2017): 438–43.

A Portrait of the Artist Using One Hand

203. god Atum, who wanks the world into existence: *The Pyramid Texts* 1248a–49, "Full Text of 'Pyramid Texts Mercer,'" n.d., https://archive.org/stream/pyramidtextsmercer/Pyramid%20Texts%20Mercer_djvu.txt.

205. The events are detailed in the Chester Beatty Papyrus I: Translation from Morgan Jerkins, "Lettuce and Kings: The Power Struggle between Horus and Set," *Michigan Quarterly Review*, https://sites.lsa.umich.edu/mqr/2015/05/lettuce-and-kings-the-power-struggle-between-horus-and-set-2.

205. sex was seen as an unremarkable activity: Charlotte Booth, *In Bed with the Ancient Egyptians* (Gloucestershire, UK: Amberley, 2015), 18.

205. held that key parts: Booth, *In Bed with the Ancient Egyptians*, 18.

206. Turin Erotic Papyrus: A. A. Shokeir and M. I. Hussein, "Sexual Life in Pharaonic Egypt: Towards a Urological View," *International Journal of Impotence Research* 16, no. 5 (2004): 385–88.

206. pornographic illustrations: Joseph A. Omlin, "Der Papyrus 55001 und seine satirisch-erotischen Zeichnungen und Inschriften," *Catalogo del Museo Egizio di Torino*, serie 1, Monumenti e testi 3 (Turin, Italy: Edizioni d'arte fratelli Pozzo, 1973).

206. popular way to deliver punchy satire: Pascal Vernus, "Stratégie d'épure et stratégie d'appogiature dans les productions dites 'artistiques' à l'usage des dominants. Le papyrus dit 'érotique' de Turin et la mise à distance des dominés," in *Art and Society: Ancient and Modern Contexts of Egyptian Art*, ed. Katalin Anna Kóthay (Budapest: Museum of Fine Arts, 2012), 116–17.

206. could have been mocking lower-class citizens: Delphine Driaux, "Toward a Study of the

Poor and Poverty in Ancient Egypt: Preliminary Thoughts," *Cambridge Archaeological Journal* 30, no. 1 (2020): 1–19.

207. "Politically motivated pornography": Lynn Hunt, "Pornography and the French Revolution," in *The Invention of Pornography: Obscenity and the Origins of Modernity 1500–1800* (New York: Zone Books, 1993), 302.

207. Marie Antoinette was portrayed: F. M. Mayeur, *L'Autrichienne en goguettes, ou l'orgie royale*, composé par un Garde-du-Corps, & publié depuis la Liberté de la Presse, & mis en musique par la Reine (Martin & Walter, 1786).

208. popular pornographic pamphlets: Peter Wagner, *Eros Revived: Erotica of the Enlightenment in England and America* (London: Paladin, 1990), 98.

208. can shape our future fantasies: *Sex, Explained*, episode 1, "Sexual Fantasies," produced by Sanya Dosani, released January 2, 2020, on Netflix.

A Short History of Erotic Literature: Or, The Awankening

209. this definition of pornography: Peter Wagner, *Eros Revived: Erotica of the Enlightenment in England and America* (London: Paladin, 1990), 7.

209. pornography today: Lynn Hunt, "Pornography and the French Revolution," in *The Invention of Pornography: Obscenity and the Origins of Modernity 1500–1800* (New York: Zone Books, 1993), 13.

210. given a name in an effort to *police*: Hunt, "Pornography and the French Revolution," 13.

210. outspoken critic of the authorities: Rictor Norton, ed., *My Dear Boy: Gay Love Letters through the Centuries* (San Francisco: Leyland, 1998).

211. sex should be spoken about by society: Pietro Aretino, "Ragionamenti," in *Aretino's Dialogues*, trans. Raymond Rosenthal (New York: Ballantine Books, 1971), 39.

213. wrath of God: Jody Greene, "Arbitrary Tastes and Commonsense Pleasures: Accounting for Taste in Cleland, Hume, and Burke," in *Launching Fanny Hill*, ed. Patsy S. Fowler and Alan Jackson (New York: AMS Press, 2003), 225.

213. he refused to vindicate his actions: John Cleland to Lovel Stanhope, law clerk in the Secretary of State's Office, November 13, 1749, quoted in Brian McCord, "'Charming and Wholesome Literature': *Fanny Hill* and the Legal Production," in *Launching Fanny Hill: Essays on the Novel and Its Influences*, ed. Patsy S. Fowler and Alan Jackson (New York: AMS Press, 2003), 277.

213. "the first original prose pornography": David Foxon, *Libertine Literature in England 1660–1745* (New York: University Books, 1965), 45.

215. "pendant around our necks": Pietro Aretino, "Lettere of 1538," *Sonetti sui sedici modi*, trans. David F. Foxon, in Foxon, *Libertine Literature in England*.

215. "pass[ed] under the Censure of being a Sodomite": Henry Merritt, "A Biographical Note on John Cleland," *Notes and Queries* 226 (1981): 305–6.

215. infer Cleland's homosexuality: George Sebastian Rousseau, *Perilous Enlightenment: Pre- and Post-Modern Discourses; Sexual, Historical* (Manchester, UK: Manchester University Press, 1991), 147.

215. "only two explicit accounts of male same-sex": Hal Gladfelder, *Fanny Hill in Bombay: The Making and Unmaking of John Cleland* (Baltimore: Johns Hopkins University Press, 2012), 9.

216. defining pornography: Commonwealth v. John Rex, No. SJC–11480 (2014), FindLaw, https://caselaw.findlaw.com/ma-supreme-judicial-court/1672119.html.

217. The justices reported: Commonwealth v. John Rex, 469 Mass. 36 (2014), http://masscases.com/cases/sjc/469/469mass36.html.

Their Eyes Were Watching Hentai

218. sexual interest in breasts: Note: The researchers didn't exclusively interview heterosexual and bisexual men; they comment that their sample was representative of the general population. Lien Holvoet et al., "Fifty Shades of Belgian Gray: The Prevalence of BDSM-Related Fantasies and Activities in the General Population," *Journal of Sexual Medicine* 14, no. 9 (2017): 1152–59.

220. smaller percentage of enslaved men: Marguerite Johnson, "The Grim Reality of the Brothels of Pompeii," *The Conversation*, December 12, 2017, https://theconversation.com/the-grim-reality-of-the-brothels-of-pompeii-88853.

221. erotic and humorous graffiti and artwork inside: *Corpus Inscriptionum Latinarum*, ed. Matteo Della Corte, vol. 4 (Berlin: Walter de Gruyter, 1955), 2175.

221. "a good fuck": Thomas A. McGinn, *The Economy of Prostitution in the Roman World* (Ann Arbor: University of Michigan Press, 2004), 162.

221. 2021: "2021 Year in Review," Pornhub, December 14, 2021, https://www.pornhub.com/insights/yir-2021.

221. 2019: "2019 Year in Review," Pornhub, December 11, 2019, https://www.pornhub.com/insights/2019-year-in-review.

222. "Human connection has become": "2021 Year in Review."

224. "quarantine" led the search on Pornhub: "2021 Year in Review."

225. a truly sizable achievement: "2019 Year in Review."

226. James Heaton and Toyoshima Mizuho: James Heaton and Toyoshima Mizuho, "Erotic Expression in Shunga," *Kyoto Journal* 18 (1991).

226. mutually beneficial experience: Danielle Talerico, "Interpreting Sexual Imagery in Japanese Prints: A Fresh Approach to Hokusai's 'Diver and Two Octopi,'" *Impressions* 23 (2001): 24–41.

227. "illegal to create a sensual scene in bed": "Toshio Maeda: Hentai Pioneer," *Tokyo Reporter*, November 8, 2008, https://www.tokyoreporter.com/japan-news/special-reports/toshio-maeda -hentai-pioneer/.

228. As writer Patrick W. Gailbraith has observed: Patrick W. Galbraith, "'The Lolicon Guy': Some Observations on Researching Unpopular Topics in Japan," in *The End of Cool Japan: Ethical, Legal, and Cultural Challenges to Japanese Popular Culture*, ed. Mark McLelland (London and New York: Routledge, 2016), 109–33.

229. "aspects of their creators' or consumers' own identities": Mark McLelland, "Australia's 'Child-Abuse Material' Legislation, Internet Regulation and the Juridification of the Imagination," *International Journal of Cultural Studies* 15, no. 5 (2011): 467–83.

229. "The distance of manga and tentacle hentai": Joel Powell Dahlquist and Lee Garth Vigilant, "Way Better Than Real: Manga Sex to Tentacle Hentai," *Net.seXXX: Readings on Sex, Pornography, and the Internet*, ed. Dennis D. Waskul (New York: Peter Lang, 2004), 91–103.

The Power of Pornography

232. shared by an increasing majority: Juliet Richters et al., "Masturbation, Paying for Sex, and Other Sexual Activities: The Second Australian Study of Health and Relationships," *Sexual Health* 11, no. 5 (2014): 461–71.

232. By 2016: Cayla Dengate, "Most People Watch Porn, but Also Agree It's Degrading to Women," *Huffington Post*, July 27, 2016, https://huffpost.com/archive/au/entry/most-people-watch-porn-but -also-agree-its-degrading-to-women_au_5cd34cf8e4b0ce845d7f13fb.

233. "general population members viewing pornography": B. Bőthe et al., "Why Do People Watch Pornography? The Motivational Basis of Pornography Use," *Psychology of Addictive Behaviors* 35, no. 2 (2021): 172–86.

233. it increases their sex drive: Vlad Burtăverde et al., "Why Do People Watch Porn? An Evolutionary Perspective on the Reasons for Pornography Consumption," *Evolutionary Psychology* 19, no. 2 (2021).

233. adds further sensory elements: Burtăverde et al., "Why Do People Watch Porn?"

233. ones that would fall under sex education: "2021 Year in Review," Pornhub, December 14, 2021, https://www.pornhub.com/insights/yir-2021.

235. **stress-motivated usage:** Bőthe et al., "Why Do People Watch Pornography?"

235. **stress-relieving methods that can develop:** Bőthe et al., "Why Do People Watch Pornography?"

235. **overconsumption of pornography:** Chris Rissel et al., "A Profile of Pornography Users in Australia: Findings from the Second Australian Study of Health and Relationships," *Journal of Sex Research* 54, no. 2 (2017): 227–40.

236. **"feeling less repressed about sex":** Rissel et al., "A Profile of Pornography Users."

236. **could improve sexual relations among adults:** Rissel et al., "A Profile of Pornography Users."

236. **big the industry of pornography has become:** Jerry Ropelato, "2006 & 2005 US Pornography Industry Revenue Statistics," TopTenReviews, 2006, accessed May 6, 2023.

236. **no sign of slowing down:** Aisha Hassan, "Porn Sites Collect More User Data Than Netflix or Hulu. This Is What They Do with It," *Quartz*, December 13, 2018, https://qz.com/1407235/porn-sites-collect-more-user-data-than-netflix-or-hulu-this-is-what-they-do-with-it/.

Index

Note: Page numbers in *italics* reference figures and tables.

About the Authors

Esmé Louise James (@Esme.Louisee) is best known for her Kinky History series on social media, where she currently has a combined following of over three million. Esmé is a PhD candidate at the University of Melbourne; her thesis investigates the emerging genre of the pornographic novel in the eighteenth century. She has written a range of articles for *The Age*, the ABC, and *The Conversation*, as well as short stories and poetry, and in 2020 she was listed in the Top 30 Emerging Writers by SBS Australia. Esmé also presents the popular *Kinky History* podcast, was a speaker at TEDxSydney in 2022, and was nominated for Best Digital Creator at the 2022 AACTA Awards.

Dr. Susan James is a senior outreach fellow in the School of Mathematics and Statistics at the University of Melbourne. She has a master of arts in mathematics from Cambridge University and a master of science and a PhD in medical statistics from the University of Leicester. With her daughter Esmé, Susan jointly created TikTok's SexTistics series, funded by Screen Australia, in 2022.